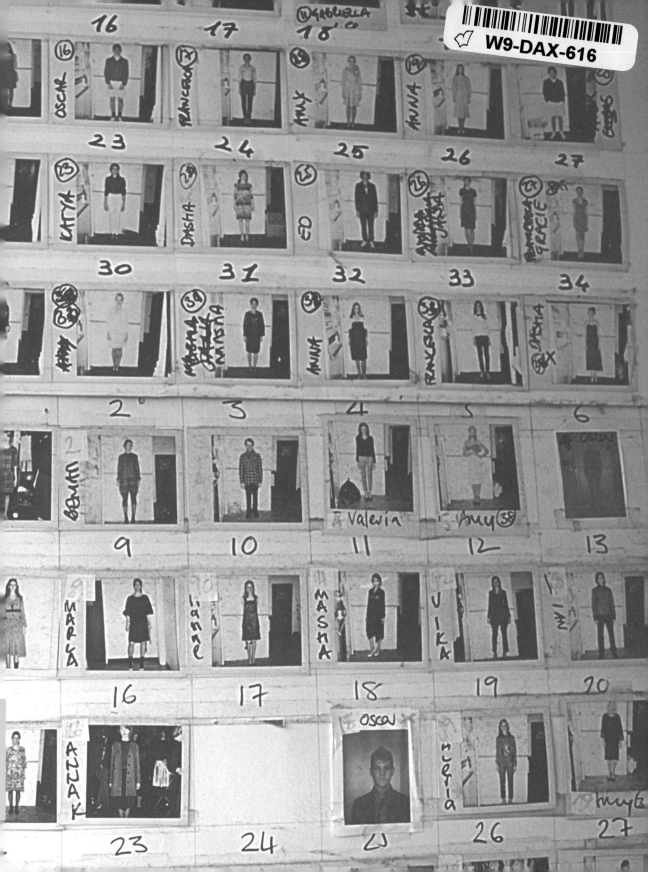

FASHION
SCANDINAVIA

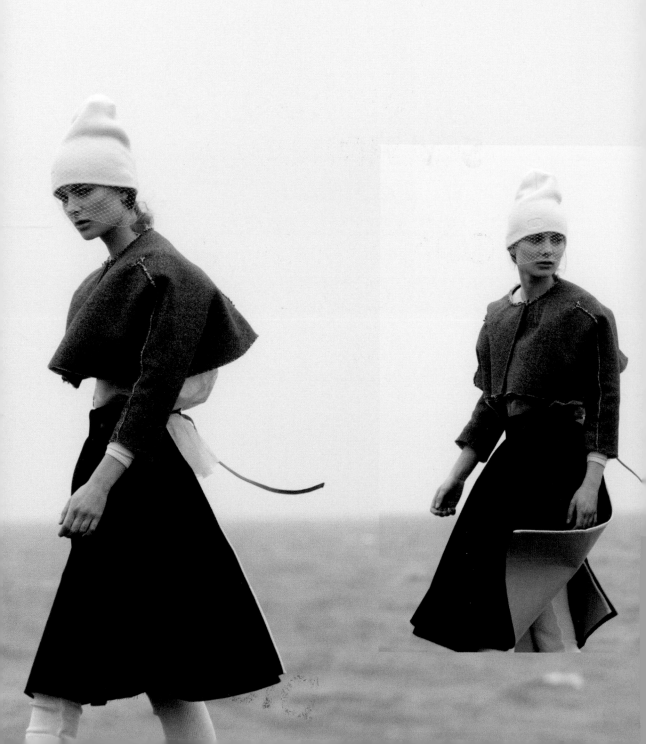

DOROTHEA GUNDTOFT

FASHION SCANDINAVIA

—

CONTEMPORARY COOL

478 illustrations, 360 in color

Thames & Hudson

**Endpapers Polaroids of runway
models in the studio of Peter Jensen.
Photo Alexander Wilson.**

p. 2 Louise Sigvardt, AW12 collection.

p. 7 Soulland, AW10 collection.

Fashion Scandinavia © 2013 Thames & Hudson Ltd, London
Text © 2013 Dorothea Gundtoft

Designed by Therese Vandling

First published in 2013 in paperback in the United States of America by
Thames & Hudson Inc., 500 Fifth Avenue, New York, New York 10110

thamesandhudsonusa.com

Library of Congress Catalog Card Number 2012944887

ISBN 978-0-500-29074-3

Printed and bound in China by Toppan Leefung

Contents

INTRODUCTION

Scandinavians have long lived and breathed design every day, from their iconic furniture and gastro food to the functional clothing they wear, which fits in with the local architecture and designed environment. The Scandinavian look is mainly characterized by simplicity, minimalism, humanized function and low-cost production. The distinctive aesthetic can be traced back to the once-dominant agricultural and fishing societies, which contributed to the clean lines and the emphasis on craftsmanship and practicality, with a palette of light tones that contrasted with the darker, richer colours of southern Europe. The style that developed was never aimed exclusively at the wealthy: it was popularized by the masses in the post-Second World War era, when social democracy came into prominence and affordable materials and ethical methods were introduced to the market. The founding of the Lunning Prize, awarded to eminent Scandinavian designers from 1951 to 1970, was also instrumental in establishing Scandinavian design as a concept.

The new matrix of social equality, tradition and industrialization heralded a major international movement. Scandinavian style attracted many consumers after *Time* magazine featured a cover image of a chair by Danish designer Hans J. Wegner in 1949. Wegner went on to win the Grand Prix at the Milan Triennale, exhibiting alongside Tapio Wirkkala of Finland and Júliana Sveinsdóttir of Iceland, marking Scandinavian design as a recognized style worldwide, originating from the five Nordic nations of Denmark, Sweden, Norway, Finland and Iceland.

It became clear that one of the outstanding features of Scandinavian style, whether in furniture or fashion, was that good design could impact positively on quality of life, notions of responsibility and social improvement. Scandinavia's emerging association with the organic also became clear, relating to Art Nouveau and running parallel alongside the Neoclassicism that was popular in the rest of Europe at the time.

Today Scandinavian fashion is a global brand. A few years ago Paris, London or New York fashion weeks would have been the big draw – the high-profile apex of the fashion calendar, due to the world-famous houses in attendance, the media presence, prestige and big budgets – but nowadays Scandinavians are also playing their part. With the additional arrival of the internet, nothing is to be missed. The time for Scandinavian clothing has come because the elements present in the designers' collections are highly in tune with the way we live and work today.

All contemporary brands want to be the first to capture a new market, while we niche consumers are keen to live and shop in a more individual and ecological way. We prefer to purchase quality items that are unique, rather than buy into 'logo mania'. It has become a statement to buy local and to choose products that have not been treated with harmful chemicals or that may not look perfect. It has also become common to incorporate these preferences within a décor that features antique or vintage furniture with modern, which is often Scandinavian. Such lifestyle choices are reflected in modern-day consumption of fashion, with shoppers buying into locally sourced or organic clothing instead of the mass-produced garments that are made in factories with poor working conditions. Scandinavians are particularly conscious of where their garments are made, and many fashion companies have signed up to ethical contracts.

The designers featured in this book represent a wide variety of approaches, but they all share a great sense of style, whether they are well-established companies with hundreds of employees and collections sold across the globe or brand-new designers just out of college but exhibiting enormous potential. Many of the designers share a common trait, which is rather minimalistic, but one also feels that they share a close-knit relationship with the fabrics they use and the quality they demand.

The texts consist either of face-to-face interviews, telephone conversations, written Q&As or my own descriptions of companies. The designers were asked to submit their own images, so that they could choose how best to present and explain their particular universe. These images are mixed with my own photo work, which has appeared in various magazines and includes backstage shots, often taken with little time and little recourse to selecting the best lens. But the equipment is not important: what counts is the story one wants to tell.

I have always been interested in finding new talent. If you have a product that is interesting and expressive, then look for people who want to promote it and seek out opportunities. If you find an unknown designer that you fall in love with, support them by buying their products. Buy local so that your designers can keep production local. Do your research and find your own style. New designers might be more expensive, but you are buying something unique. In addition, you will feel as if he or she is designing for you exclusively … and that is luxury.

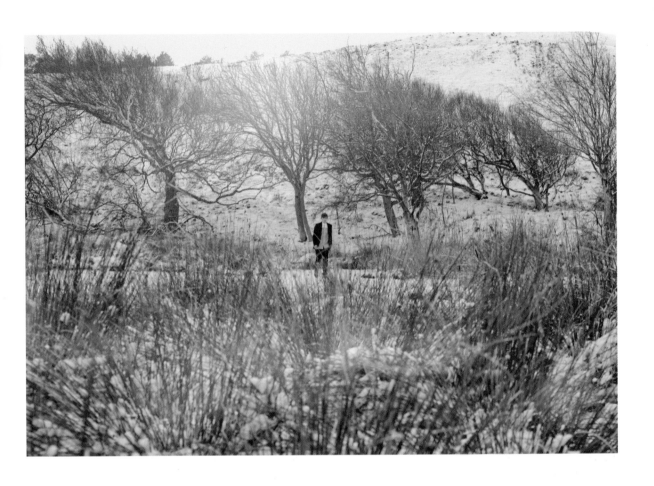

'The time for Scandinavian clothing
has come because the elements present in
the designers' collections are highly in tune
with the way we live and work today'

5PREVIEW

THIS SWEDISH BRAND MAY GIVE THE IMPRESSION OF BEING A SMALL T-SHIRT DIY,
BUT, EVEN IF FOUNDER EMELI MÅRTENSSON LOVES THAT APPROACH, HER COLLECTIONS
ARE IN FACT SOLD ALL OVER THE WORLD. IN HER CAMPAIGNS SHE HAS FEATURED
THE EX-HARPER'S BAZAAR FASHION EDITOR LINDA RODIN, AND HER
DESIGNS HAVE BEEN WORN BY THE LIKES OF P. DIDDY.

Tell me about your upbringing and where you are from. I'm from the south of Sweden, but I moved to Italy straight after high school to study industrial design at Accademia Italiana in Florence. I stayed there for ten years (with a little break when I moved back to Stockholm to study graphic design and copywriting at Forsbergs). I studied fashion design for a year at Istituto Europeo di Design in Milan, and I spent a couple of months at a private academy for pattern making. Then I got headhunted for Miss Sixty and worked there as a print designer and illustrator for five years. I've always drawn, but I think it was during my fashion studies that I really started to find my own style, thanks to a great Dutch teacher. He taught me that if I'm not capable of drawing a straight line it's fine anyway, and so I found my own personal style.

How and why did you start your company? I started 5PREVIEW as a 'hobby', printing T-shirts at home at night. I've always been into DIY and I loved the idea of a simple minimalistic product – it probably comes from my Scandinavian background – compared to Italy, the centre of bling-bling and rhinestones and embroideries and stuff. Thanks to the use of Myspace at the time, 5PREVIEW got a lot of attention on the internet and that put the product straight into the right shops around the world.

Where does your main inspiration come from? Anything Scandinavian, or mostly from outside? After Italy I moved to New York and then back to Sweden. I love the fresh air here, the awareness of the people (of all kinds – trends, culture, fashion, film, music, books, recycling, ambience, etc.), the politeness, and most of all the ability to live on an island surrounded by the sea but in the centre of a capital. So the calm here inspires me a lot.

It's easy to focus. I love nature and how easy it is to reach it. I think inspiration comes from hard work, so this is the perfect place to get inspired and to work. I travel a lot and that helps, too (I love Japan!).

What is your first step when you design a collection? I do a lot of watercolour sketches of all the stuff I really want in the collection. I put them on a wall and start to organize them into fabric groups, etc.

I love the image of Linda Rodin in a room full of objects. Tell me how it relates to your universe. It's a typical example of how 5PREVIEW interacts with other creative people. Those pictures were made in a collaboration with a New York-based photographer, Paola Ambrosi de Magistris. She got a box of clothes from our last collection and could interpret them in her own way. Working as a photographer in New York you meet a lot of people, and she met Linda Rodin on another shoot. Linda is the ex-fashion editor of *Harper's Bazaar*, ex-model, now stylist, and promotes her own beauty product brand. In the pictures she styled herself with the clothes from our SS12 collection, 'SHORELINE'. It's great. It's shot in her apartment. We published it in our magazine, *5-PIECE-PAPER n° 4*, together with other similar collaborations. It's an ongoing project that really gives me a lot of satisfaction.

Where do you produce your T-shirts and garments? I started out with the 'Made In Italy' handprinted T-shirts, then it became too much to print everything by hand. Requests grew, so we moved the whole production to China. Now, slowly, we're trying to get it back to Europe again. All the knitwear and belts are 'Made In Italy'.

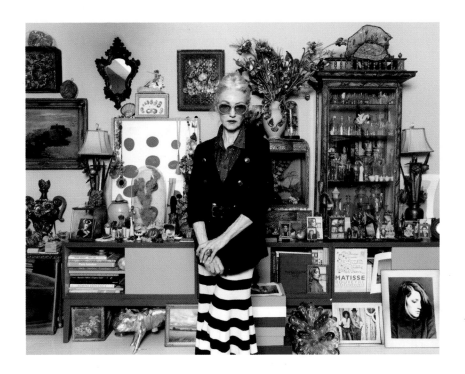

<u>Above and right:</u> Stylist Linda
Rodin at home in New York,
wearing 5PREVIEW.

<u>Below:</u> Illustrator and
5PREVIEW collaborator Ragnar
Persson, wearing an original
Joy Division T-shirt.

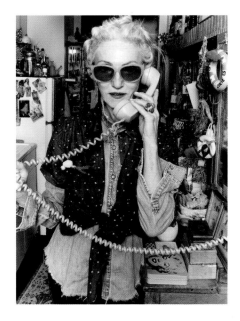

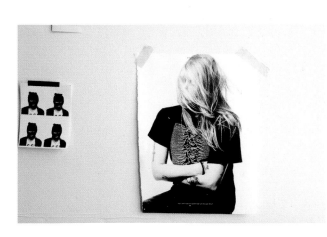

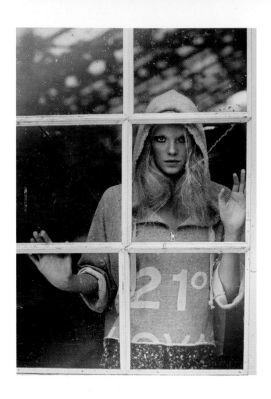

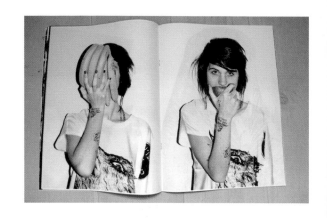

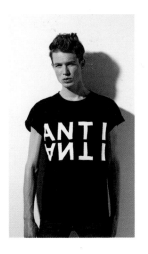

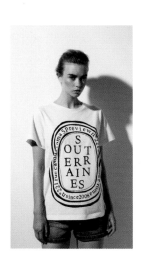

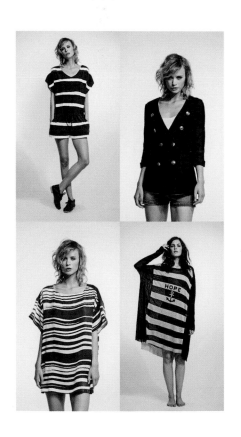

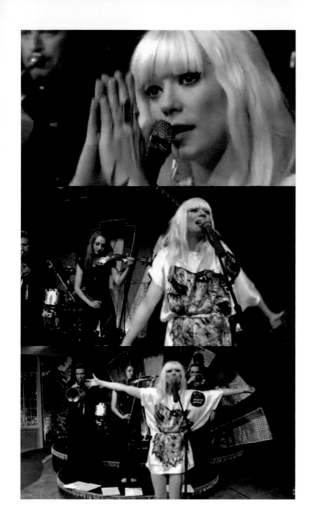

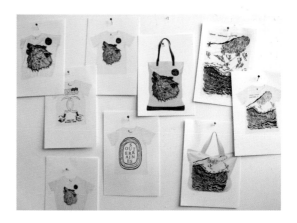

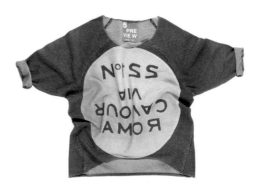

Left: Video stills featuring singer Mieze Katz wearing a 5PREVIEW silk dress with LUPO print designed by Ragnar Persson.

You have also created the clothes for videos. Tell me about those projects. 5PREVIEW clothes have been in several videos – for the Italian artist Bugo, for Black Acid (Richard Fearless from Death in Vegas's new project), Swedish NonTiq and, last but not least, the P. Diddy video, 'Dirty Money'.

Where are you sold outside of Scandinavia? Our largest market is Italy; after that Asia (mainly Japan) and Germany.

We also work with distributors in the US, Russia, Australia, Spain and the UK. Our Scandinavian market is completely based in Denmark, where we sell in more than forty stores. Sweden is still new ground for us – strange, isn't it? – but we are going to work actively on sales here, together with Örjan Andersson (founder of Cheap Monday and now new brand Örjan Andersson, for which 5PREVIEW helps out with the graphics).

ACNE

THIS SWEDISH MULTI-BRAND ORIGINATES FROM A COLLECTIVE BASED
AROUND THE IDEAS OF JONNY JOHANSSON AND THREE COLLEAGUES. IN 1996,
THE TEAM CREATED A LIFESTYLE ALL-ROUNDER. THEIR AIM WAS TO COMBINE ART AND
FASHION WITH ADVERTISING AND FILM. TODAY THE COMPANY IS AN ELITE
SCANDINAVIAN BRAND, WITH A GREAT MARKETING STRATEGY, WHICH
HAS TAKEN THE ONE-TIME JEANS COMPANY TO NEW HEIGHTS.

Acne started life in 1996 as a collective, with its founders based in the fields of graphic design, television production and advertising. They had the idea of distributing one hundred pairs of unisex jeans with bright red stitching to family and friends. Inspired by the Warhol Factory era, they – like Andy – must have had the right friends, as soon all the cognoscenti of Stockholm and the rest of Sweden wanted more from this brand with the strange name. But Acne is not just a skin disease: it's also an acronym for 'Ambition to Create Novel Expressions'.

Jonny Johansson functions as the overall creative director. He takes inspiration mostly from furniture, architecture, artists including Jean Cocteau, and travel to cities such as New York. The spirit of the company, meanwhile, is inspired by simple, minimalistic, clean lines and Scandinavian furniture from the 1920s and '30s.

The extremely busy team travels the world, as the brand now spans multiple areas – from clothing to furniture and toys. It has shops in all the right locations, including Greene Street in New York; Le Marais in Paris; Paddington, Sydney; and Antwerp in Belgium. Edgy shop openings have attracted stellar attendees such as Daphne Guinness.

Acne also has a production company, specializing in film and digital. They have produced ad campaigns for H&M, Jaguar, IKEA and Canon, to name but a few. They have also made documentaries and a TV series on fashion called *Streetsmart*. In addition the company publishes the periodical, *Acne Paper*.

Collaborations with the likes of Lanvin often come about by chance (Jonny Johansson happened to meet the designer Alber Elbaz at a dinner). Acne have also collaborated with the magazine *Fantastic Man* to create a pair of gentleman's jeans, and they have worked on a line of sofas inspired by the furniture designer Carl Malmsten. Other collaborations include work with Bianchi Bicycles, the jewelers Michael Zobel and Husam El Odeh, and Swarowski.

Jonny Johansson has stated that fashion isn't art, but he can't live without both. The photographer Lord Snowdon has participated in a touring exhibition of sixty images edited by his daughter, Frances von Hofmannsthal, featuring well-known personalities and Acne shirts. The company has also showcased sculptures by Helmut Lang in its shop on Dover Street in London.

Acne works with the Fair Wear Foundation. This ensures that the process of production is responsible. The company also only collaborates with manufacturers who have signed up to the foundation's Corporate Social Responsibility contract.

As one of the first Scandinavian brands with their own stand-alone catwalk show at both Paris and London fashion weeks, Acne understands how to invite the right fashion crowd, throw amazing parties with great concepts (such as having their waiters wear floral headpieces), and produce minimalistic clothing – all within a highly sought-after universe that is specifically designed to promote art and to reflect Scandinavian values.

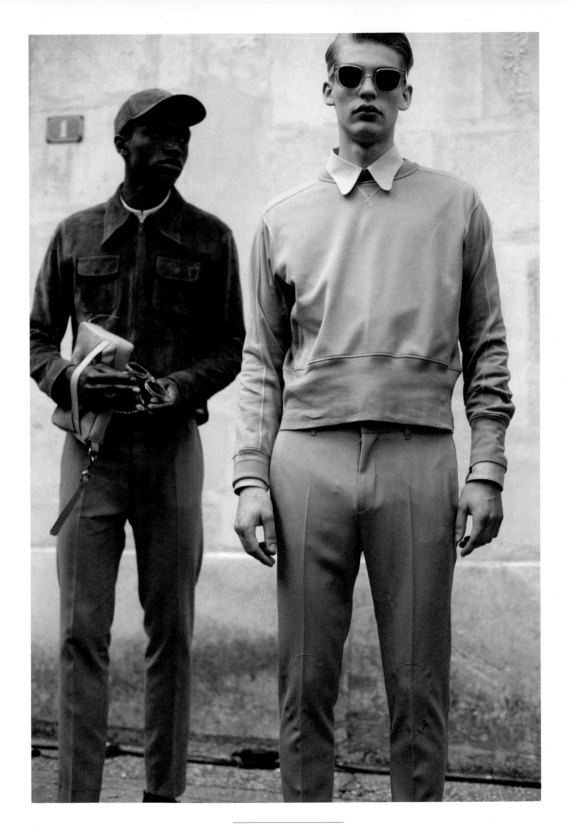

Below: Acne shop
in Copenhagen.

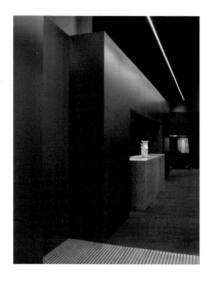

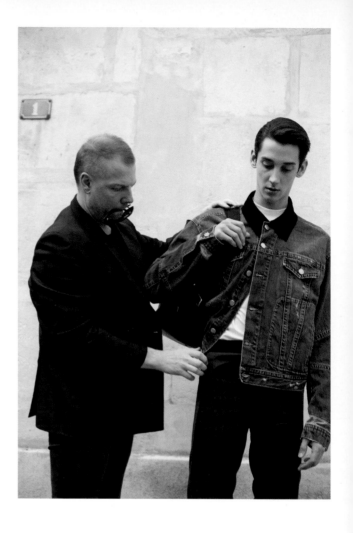

Right: Founder Jonny
Johansson at a fitting.

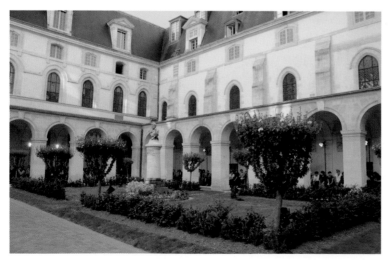

Left: Show during
Paris Fashion Week.

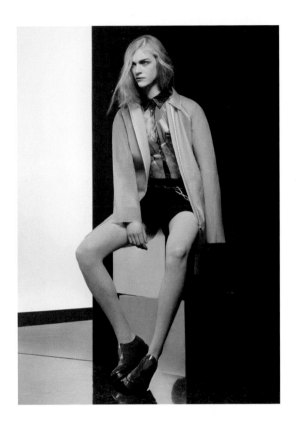

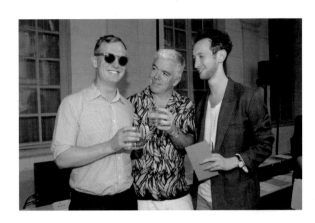

Below: Acne shop in Paris.

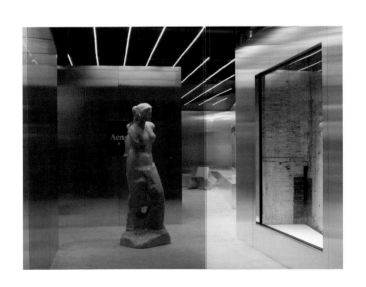

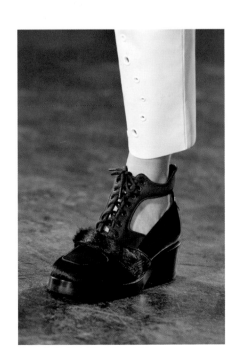

ALTEWAI.SAOME

THE TWO YOUNG SWEDISH DESIGNERS NATALIA ALTEWAI AND
RANDA SAOME FOUNDED THEIR COMPANY IN 2009. THEIR COLLECTIONS OFTEN
INCLUDE GARMENTS THAT ARE CUSTOM-MADE AND TAILORED. THE PAIR OPENED
STOCKHOLM FASHION WEEK IN JANUARY 2012 AND ALREADY HAVE A PROMISING
FUTURE AT THE FOREFRONT OF EDGY SCANDINAVIAN DESIGN.

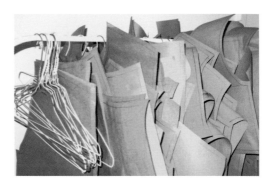

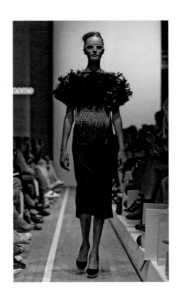

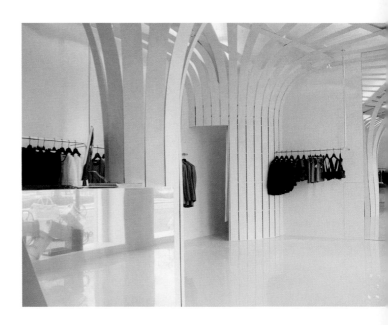

<u>Right:</u> Patriksson
Communication in Stockholm,
showcasing Altewai.Saome.

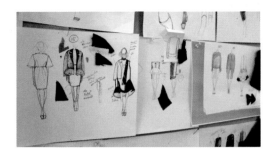

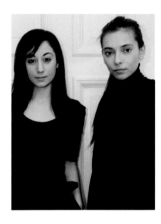

Above: Designers Randa
Saome and Natalia Altewai.

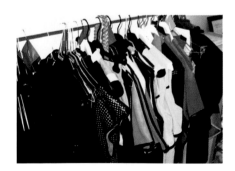

Tell me about the beginning of your brand. We started talking about creating our own brand while we were still studying in Milan. After our studies we both began working in Italy but soon decided that it was time for us to go back to Sweden. It was now or never; all or nothing.

Who did you work for in Italy? Natalia worked for Etro and I worked for an embroidery company.

You are both so young and the brand already looks very 'international'! Where does this eye for detail come from? When we were in school, our teachers always encouraged us to experiment with fabrics and different materials and to add details to our collections. We have always been very interested in working with details, such as embroidery, which for us make the garments interesting and exciting.

The garments seem quite complicated to manufacture, like pieces of art. How do you go about achieving them? The heavy embroidered pieces we produce only by request, and they are tailor-/custom-made.

There seems to be a lot of embroidery on your garments, like in a French couture house, but, since you don't have the staff, who creates these magnificent pieces? We design all the embroideries ourselves and send the final designs to a company that produces them. But it has also happened that we have done embroideries ourselves by hand for our shows.

Where does your inspiration come from? Usually it's a feeling we follow. It can literally be anything, but we always keep the strong, confident woman in mind.

You started in 2009. How has the process of developing a collection changed? It hasn't changed at all. We've done four collections and thus far the process is the same.

Now you live in Malmö. Do you get inspired by the city or do you go to Copenhagen a lot, or do you mostly travel? We do live in Malmö but sometimes it actually feels as if we live only in our office. We spend many hours there, which leaves us with no time to get inspired by the city. We do travel a lot to Copenhagen, Milan and Paris for work, and the feeling of those cities is always inspiring.

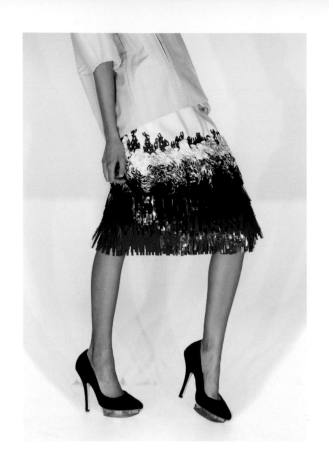

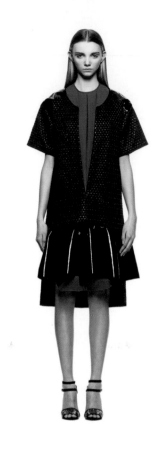

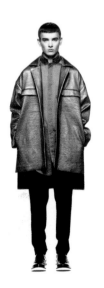

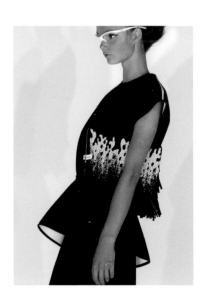

'We have always been
interested in working
with details, such as
embroidery, which
for us make garments
interesting and exciting'

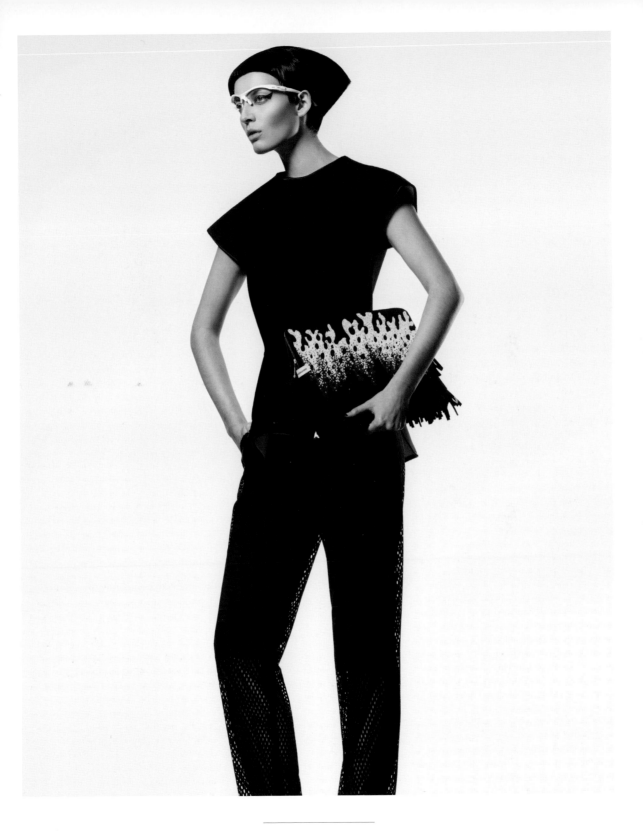

ANN-SOFIE BACK

SHE IS STILL FEATURED ON THE CENTRAL SAINT MARTINS WEBSITE,
NEXT TO ALEXANDER MCQUEEN, EVEN THOUGH SHE GRADUATED IN 1998.
THE SWEDISH DESIGNER PRESENTS HER COLLECTIONS DURING LONDON FASHION WEEK,
WITH REVIEWS FROM THE LIKES OF VOGUE, WHO RECOGNIZE HER TALENT FOR SHOCKING
AUDIENCES WITH INSPIRATION TAKEN FROM SUBJECTS INCLUDING PORNOGRAPHY, CARS
AND MURDER SCENES. IN ADDITION TO HEADING THE LABELS ANN-SOFIE BACK ATELJE
AND BACK, ANN-SOFIE IS THE CREATIVE DIRECTOR AT CHEAP MONDAY
AND COLLABORATES WITH TOPSHOP AND FRED PERRY.

You graduated from Central Saint Martins in 1998. It must have been different back then. How did you experience the atmosphere? I was the first Swede to graduate from the MA course and I had no idea of what to expect. Coming from the Swedish educational system, where pupils constantly question and criticize the tutors, I was taken aback by the level of respect and fear that ruled at Central Saint Martins. I think it was naivety that got me through.

Before you started your own brand did you work for different designers? Margareta van den Bosch at H&M gave me my first design job, working extra hours during studies, and I also spent a couple of years at Acne back in the days when it was only Jonny [Johansson; see p. 12] and me in the design team.

It only took a few years, though, for you to debut with a ready-to-wear collection at the Purple institute in Paris. Did you feel that Paris was a better platform for your designs than Scandinavia? Scandinavia wasn't an option back then, and I was based in London full-time. I felt at the time that my designs corresponded better with the Parisian aesthetic.

I remember seeing a show of yours in Copenhagen, and also a presentation in London that I covered backstage. You seemed to have a lot of focus and a very strong presence. Did you always know you were going to be leading teams? I know what I want and I'm organized. Since I can't do patterns or sew, I quickly had to learn how to delegate.

Your work has also been featured in art shows at the V&A Museum in London and the Palais de Tokyo in Paris, among others. Do you see your designs as wearable pieces of art, or do you prefer to combine those aspects? I never felt the need to distinguish between whether what I did was art or fashion, though when asked I said fashion. Art doesn't interest or fascinate me the way fashion does. I find fashion far more important and difficult. Today I wouldn't hesitate to say it was fashion — no question about it.

This brings to mind the themes of your collections, which have included porn, the punk DIY aesthetic, plastic surgery, the cult of celebrity, etc. But even though the theme might sound vulgar your design is always very streamlined. It could be an office woman wearing it or an editor at a fashion week... I need to use inspiration that disturbs me. It's often social or cultural phenomena I don't agree with that end up as themes for the collections. For the AW 12 collection we started out with the theme 'God'. I can't stand any religion, and during the course of designing we realized we didn't have any relationship with God at all, so we ended up with the Scandinavian concept of 'Jante's Law', a set of rules that basically tell you that you are crap. Look it up!

I know about it, since I'm Danish. It's very ugly! But when you decide that a collection is to have a strong theme, you must have a reason for wanting to express it through garments. It's more for me — to keep my interest in the collection during the process — than for public

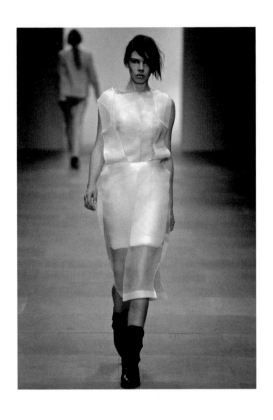

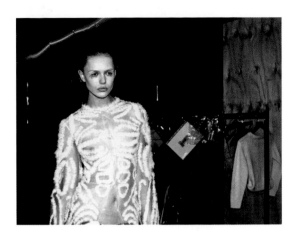

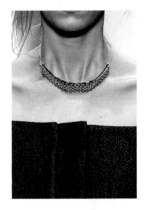

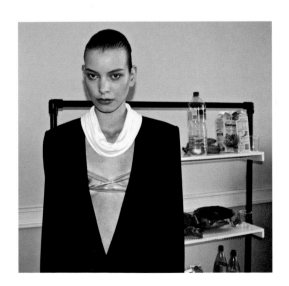

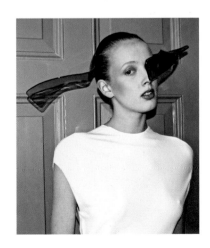

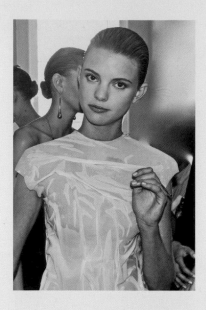

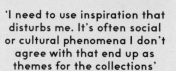

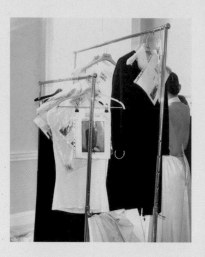

'I think it was naivety that got me through'

ON FASHION STUDIES

'I need to use inspiration that disturbs me. It's often social or cultural phenomena I don't agree with that end up as themes for the collections'

ON INSPIRATION

'Art doesn't interest or fascinate me the way fashion does. I find fashion far more important and difficult'

ON ART AND FASHION

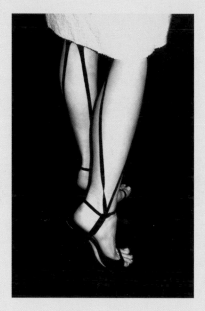

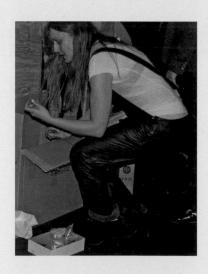

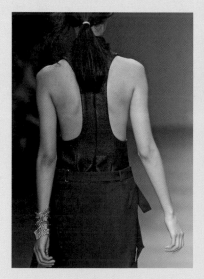

Left: Designer Ann-Sofie Back.

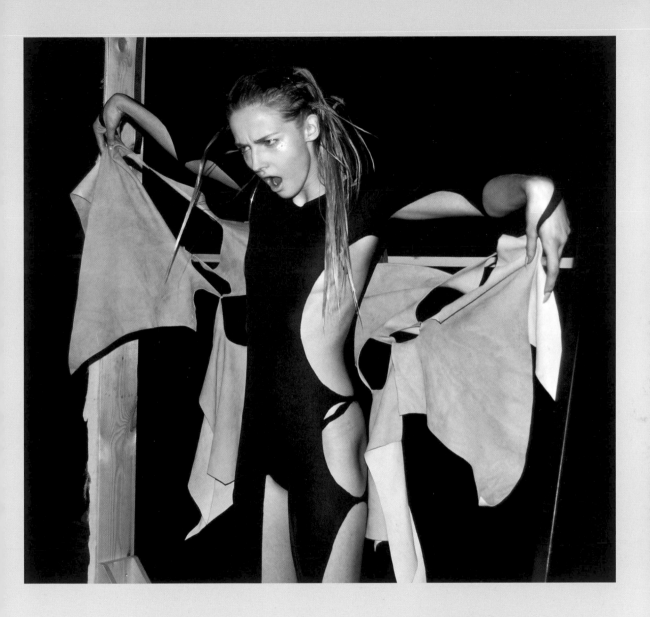

consumption. It justifies what I do, in my own regard. That's my point of difference and my excuse for continuing.

What is your plan for the next five years? Do you want to stay in Sweden, move out, expand your brand, do more consultancy, more styling? I spend 50% of my time on my own company, which suits me fine since I have amazing staff. I have also taken over as the sole creative director of design at Cheap Monday. I truly enjoy my work there and I'm learning an awful lot. With BACK we are concentrating on Scandinavia and Benelux, and Ann-Sofie Back Atelje is looking into expanding its accessories line.

ANNE SOFIE MADSEN

SHE HAD JUST GRADUATED FROM DESIGN SCHOOL IN DENMARK WHEN
SHE WAS CHOSEN FOR THE OFFICIAL OPENING SHOW OF COPENHAGEN FASHION
WEEK 2011. THINGS HAVE BEEN MOVING FAST FOR THIS DESIGNER, AND SHE HAS ALREADY
BEEN NOTICED BY AMERICAN VOGUE'S HAMISH BOWLES, WHO COMMENTED:
'AN IMPRESSIVE RUNWAY DEBUT FOR A DESIGNER WHOSE WORK EXPERIENCES
WITH GALLIANO AND MCQUEEN HAVE CLEARLY PAID DIVIDENDS.'

You have done impressively well in just one year, or how long is it since you have been independent? I started my own practice in 2010 and showed during London Fashion Week as part of Vauxhall Fashion Scout's 'Ones to Watch' show in February the same year. In 2011 I opened Copenhagen Fashion Week and started my ready-to-wear production.

How did all this media frenzy begin, with everyone wanting to know more about you … although it's not so weird since your pieces are absolutely beautiful and not the easy ready-to-wear type? I think the press became aware of my designs after my MA graduation collection. The collection was featured in some powerful media, which brought a lot of attention from both the Danish and international press.

Is everything handmade? If so, how many people does that take, since some of the pieces seem so delicate and others are print? Many of our garments require a lot of hand-sewing and drapery. We do half of the collection as made-to-measure, which means that it is built on a mannequin and sewn by hand. For the rest of the collection, we make the first pieces here, but then send them elsewhere for production when they have to go to the shops. Regarding the prints, I usually start by creating the pattern for the garment. Then I start painting the illustration with watercolour and pencil. Finally, both are scanned and edited further in Photoshop. After finalizing the creation process, I choose the fabric. Then I source the material and send the digital files of both print and pattern for production. The production of the print involves using a multicoloured printing method (instead of spot colours, as with screenprinting). For the dresses, we normally work on stretch silk chiffon or invisible tulle as the basis. But from there the techniques and methods used vary a lot for each design. When creating a collection, I spend approximately three months with a team consisting of around eight interns.

How long does it take? Some garments take two months to produce, while others only take two days. However, during the whole collection creation process, everything is a work in progress, as we keep on trying out techniques, compositions and mixes of materials. For instance, on the skeleton trousers from AW12/13, we first used quilted silk and pleated cotton, then we tried an artificial material, but ended up doing them in flat leather … before finally deciding to do them in moulded leather. Afterwards we chose a silver finish, but then changed it to a black finish. For me, creating a piece for a collection is not about thinking of a garment, but about thinking of an expression within a shape, material or colour. I learned this from being a student and having to express shapes that had to convey a message. It was a very inspiring but also abstract way to learn how to use materials. Now, I always try to give interns an opportunity to see the process of different methods of creation. Another example for this collection is the frills that you can find on most of the garments. Aligned with the 'Sedna' storyline, we wanted to create ready-to-wear and made-to-measure garments that were inspired by traditional Inuit costumes, so we searched for inspiration in the patterns that they used for their beading. However, in order to make the design more modern and to have a more futuristic take on it, we used shiny plastic material from the Danish furniture manufacturer Kvadrat. We organized a pattern for the frills and added pleated, sandwashed silk for a softer expression.

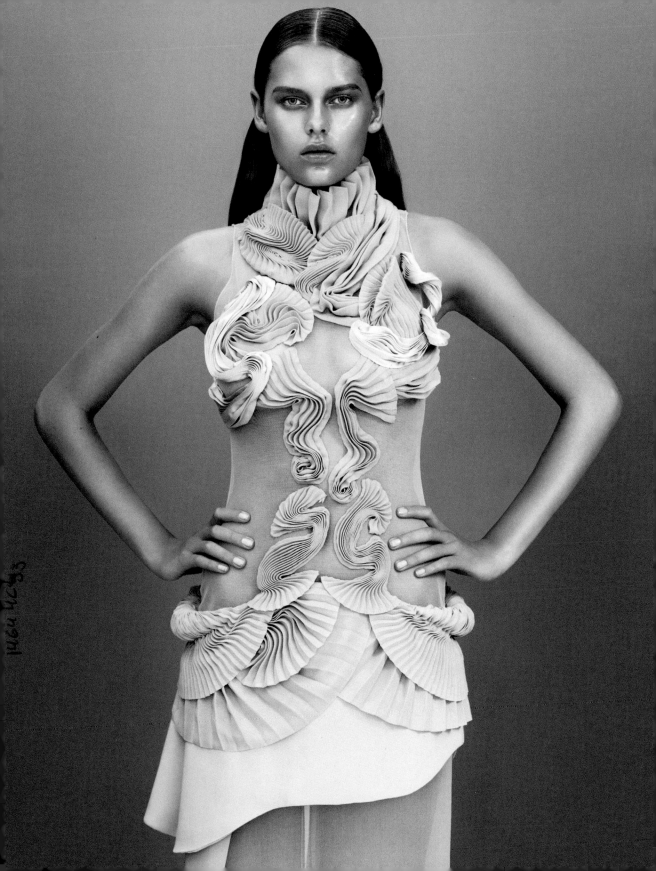

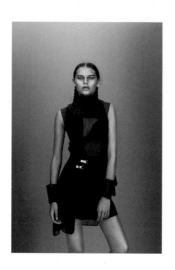

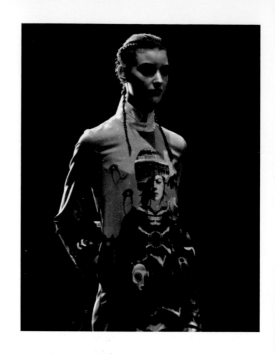

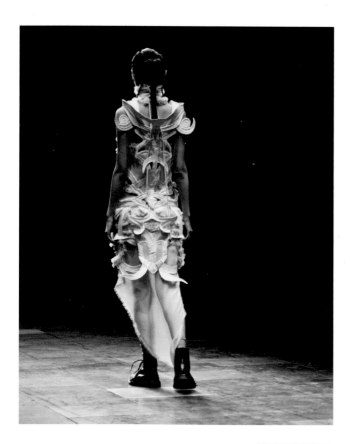

'I figured I might as well have my own name at the back of the blouse'

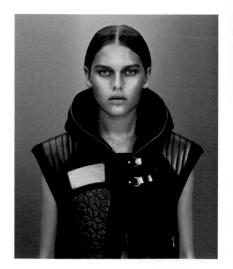

How do you have time to sit down and draw illustrations? If I have to draw something, I have to zone out into my own world, but I can't do that if I have to do paperwork and manage a team, deadlines, shows, everything. How do you manage? I actually prefer to work in noisy places. I'm just more productive in a productive place. For me drawing is the focal point, so in a way it has changed from being something I could do when all the other things were done into being something I need to do before starting on anything else. When the press covered my MA graduation collection, they also showed many of my drawings and after that I was contacted by publishers who asked me to do illustrations for various projects – and since then I've had four books published. Regarding the management of time and resources, I have a business partner, Simon, who takes care of all the commercial matters so that I can focus solely on the creative part.

Tell me about your time in Paris and London. I moved to Paris and started looking for an internship. I think I was chosen by John Galliano mainly because of my illustration portfolio. I mostly did illustrations there, but I also hand-painted flowers on silk for the showpieces. I was there for ten months, during which I learned about Galliano's different way of working. Key learning points were 3D fabric manipulation, beadwork and hand-embroidery, which I wasn't really aware of before working in Paris. Elisa Palomino, my boss at Galliano, then recommended me to the recruitment agency Floriane de Saint Pierre, and through them I got a job at Alexander McQueen as a junior designer. During my time there I learned a lot about working with an atelier – production and so on – and I became aware of my wish to create collections of my own. I think that

being a junior designer for twelve months, and working from 8 in the morning until 2 after midnight every day, made me realize that I actually wanted to have my own business. I figured, if I'm going to work like this I might as well have my own name at the back of the blouse.

You studied at the Royal Danish Academy of Fine Arts School of Design. Would you recommend that instead of the obvious Central Saint Martins? Would you recommend people trying to find alternative ways? It's obvious that you don't get as much press when you graduate from a Danish school as when you graduate from Central Saint Martins. I really enjoyed studying in Denmark, but, if I were to recommend anything for others, I would recommend Central Saint Martins as it would have made a lot of things easier. The brand value and reputation of the school give more opportunities, although I think people often believe that if you go to a famous design school then everything just comes automatically.

What would you say if you had to explain to someone who is studying at a design school and trying to be where you are now, what you did and how it was possible? I think it's important to get as much as possible out of your studies and to do internships, while also being determined and developing a very good work ethic.

Where do you see your brand expanding? What is your dream? I would like to transform couture techniques for ready-to-wear, while also having a profitable business. I would like for others to share my vision, and I would like to expand my brand globally.

'For me, creating a piece for a collection is about thinking of an expression within a shape, material or colour'

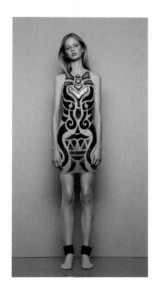

Below and opposite:
Illustrations by
Anne Sofie Madsen.

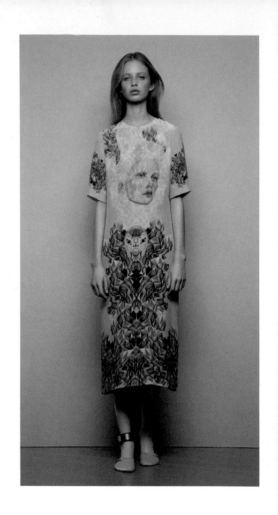

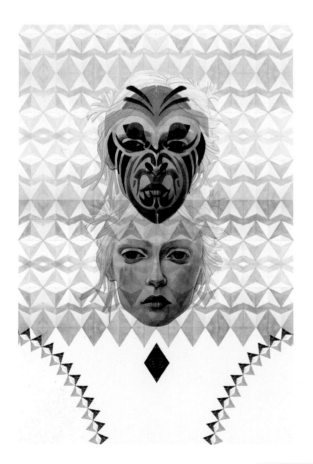

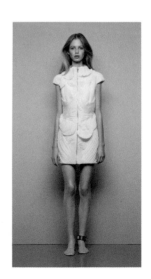

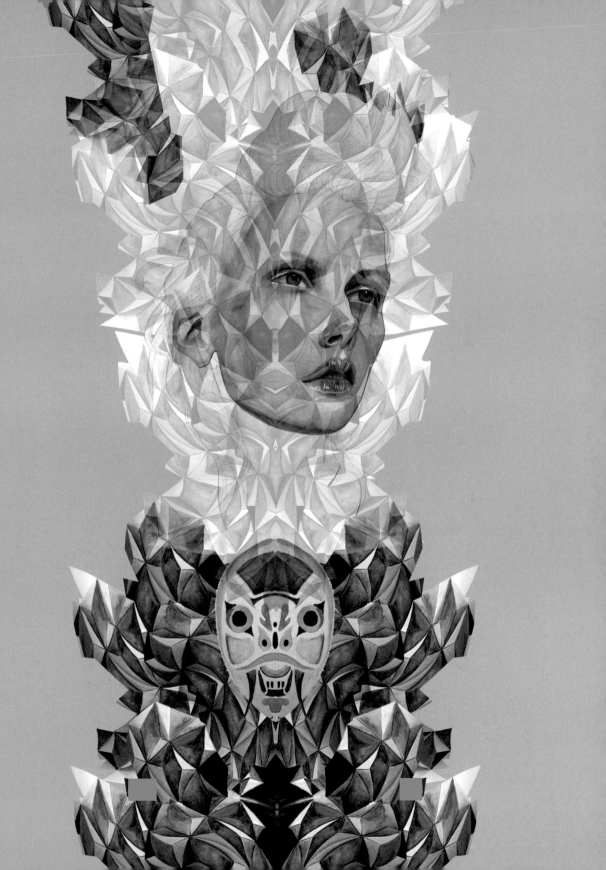

ASGER JUEL LARSEN

HE GREW UP SKATEBOARDING BUT WAS SECRETLY KNITTING WITH HIS MOTHER
AND ATTENDING EXHIBITIONS. THIS TALENTED YOUNG DESIGNER FROM DENMARK,
EDUCATED AT LONDON COLLEGE OF FASHION, HAD A SUCCESSFUL START TO HIS LABEL
BY PRESENTING IT DURING LONDON AND COPENHAGEN FASHION WEEKS.
HIS COLLECTIONS HAVE APPEARED IN THE HIPPEST PLACES, INCLUDING
THE LONDON CONCEPT STORE MACHINE-A.

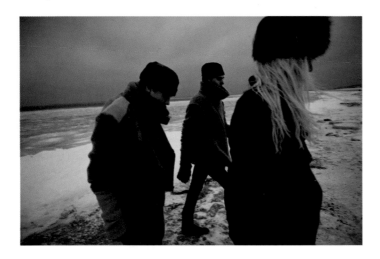

'I've come to the
conclusion that almost
every collection I've
done has a starting
point in my youth'

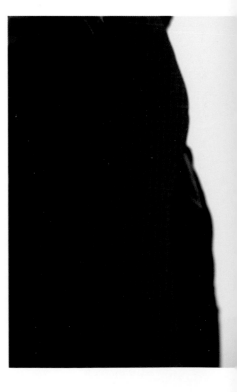

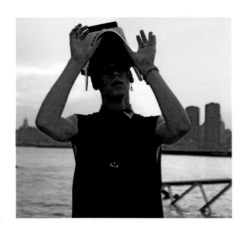

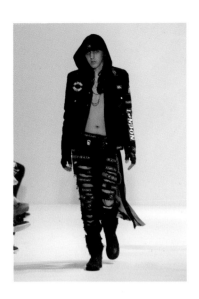

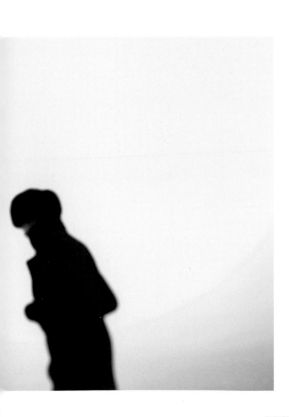

Tell me where your inspiration comes from when you design. I've been asking myself that for some time! Basically I've come to the conclusion that almost every collection I've done has a starting point in my youth – how I grew up, what toys I played with, my time as a skateboarder… I also had a close friend who was a goth. At the time I never realized what it really meant, just that I was attracted to the mysterious, dark shadow that surrounded him and his friends. That being said, the mixture has to occur, and that's why I think it's necessary also to draw inspiration from something entirely different. For me this is the history of war, and in particular military tailoring and shape. The madness comes alive from my youth and the structure arrives from my interest in warfare.

What was your upbringing like, and where did you study design? I would say I had a pretty unrestricted upbringing, with a lot of love. I could have become whatever I wanted and my family would have been supportive. The women on my mother's side of the family all did something in relation to textiles, whether it was embroidery, hand-knitting or sewing. I learned that at an early age, but it wasn't until later that I realized it was my 'calling'. Also I couldn't really tell my skater friends that I was sitting and knitting with my mother when I wasn't hanging out with them! I did my BA in menswear at London College of Fashion and thought I was going to work at some colossal fashion house after graduating. Luckily my BA collection was well received and that pretty much kickstarted the idea of having my own label. That same summer I got a scholarship to do my MA at London College of Fashion, and that was convenient because I was then able to do smaller collections outside college and still keep awareness of my label while finishing my MA.

You are also very active at nighttime. How do you have time to work on collections? Do you ever sleep?! I live my life in periods measured around each collection. By that I mean that when I work on a new collection I do nothing but work, work and work. I get deeply involved and it almost becomes a personal state of mind. I don't want any obstacles or disruptions from the outside world. After showing, I go Cuban: I break free and I clear my mind. Almost all my friends do music, so they often help me by inviting me to join them wherever they're booked to play. And then after some time I move on to the next collection.

You present your collection during London Fashion Week and now also at Copenhagen. Tell me about these different experiences and what they give you.

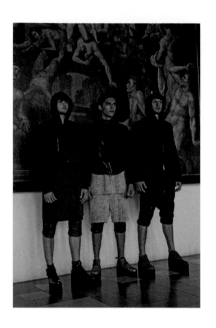

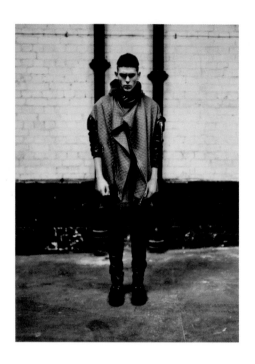

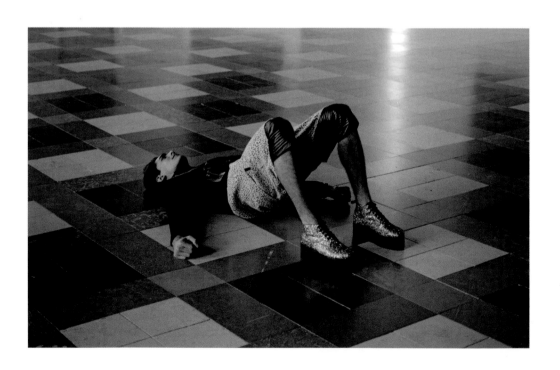

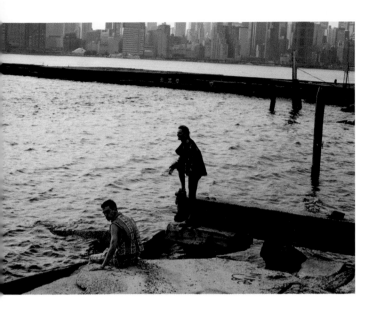

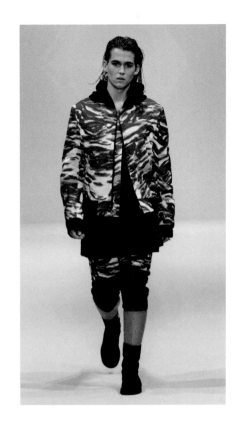

'I want to pursue making new collections that are creative and imaginative as well as wearable'

London is where the label is based and it has shaped me into the designer I am today. Last season I showed back home for the first time and the experience was overwhelming. When you've been away from your home country for almost five years and you return to display what you've accomplished, it has to be good. We got the chance to do a show at the National Museum of Denmark. That was emotional for me because my mother used to take me there almost every month when I was growing up. It's one of the prettiest places in Copenhagen and the support was great. More than 1,200 people turned up and I was really pleased with the show.

Where is your collection sold now? It's sold in Copenhagen, Tokyo, Shanghai, New York, Florence, Hamburg, Berlin and Stockholm. We're also going to have a show in London and we'll take part in a showroom in Paris.

What do you want to develop your brand into? Any strategies? I want to see it grow steadily, as it has up until now, with a more thorough and professional approach, and I want to pursue making new collections that are creative and imaginative as well as wearable. And maybe one day we'll expand and do womenswear.

ASTRID ANDERSEN

SHE IS A NEWCOMER TO THE SCANDINAVIAN FASHION SCENE
BUT NOT TO MAGAZINES SUCH AS i-D AND VOGUE ITALIA, WHO HAVE
FOLLOWED HER SINCE HER GRADUATION FROM LONDON'S ROYAL COLLEGE OF ART.
BASED IN COPENHAGEN, SHE OPERATES WITH SUPPORT FROM THE BRITISH
FASHION COUNCIL AND FUNDING FROM FASHION EAST. SHE IS
ONE OF THE MOST PROMISING MENSWEAR DESIGNERS
ACTIVE IN SCANDINAVIA TODAY.

You did your MA in menswear at the Royal College of Art. Tell me about your experience there. I have heard it is very tough! I graduated in 2010 and it was a real privilege to be able to study at the RCA. You meet people who are incredibly skilled and amazing at pushing your potential to the fullest. It's hard work and you learn how to deal with criticism and opinions, and when to put your heart and soul into your work and when to step away from it to make it better.

What happened after you finished your MA? I went to Trieste as part of the 'ITS#NINE' competition, and later on to Milan as part of *Vogue* Italia's 'Talent 2010' exhibition. After that there was a comedown and four months of not really knowing what to do. I had two big job interviews but had already received orders for my graduate collection. I was also approached by Harrods to be part of their talent platform, but that required a re-make of my graduate collection and at that point I was really ready to do something new, so the thought of making a new collection for AW11 came along.

You have had a lot of press coverage. Have you been working hard in that area, or did you let your PR do all the work? I think I generally make pieces that are very suited for the press. My work has a show factor and a sense of something young and playful both in shape and colour. I do also have an amazing PR in London, Ella Dror, who really does a lot to keep me in the race.

Where did you meet Ella Dror? I met her right after my graduate show at the RCA, when she was involved in a PR/shop in Soho in London and was on her way to setting up her own PR company. She immediately believed in my design aesthetic, and has continued to do so ever since.

You won the Brioni Creativity and Innovation Award at the RCA. I have heard about the trip to Italy where you stay at their little castle and see how they work up close. What did you design for them? We had to design a traveller's jacket – an iconic Brioni piece that holds about a hundred pockets! So I created a travelling vagabond whose pockets were massive and outgrowing him. For me it was more a fun and conceptual project, and my first ever experimentation with fur.

Do you live in London today or Copenhagen? Where is the brand based? Today I live in Copenhagen, but I am in London at least once a month. Mine is now a British brand (though the manufacturing is run from Copenhagen), mainly because of all the amazing support I get from the British Fashion Council and Fashion East.

Do you get your fabrics and production done in Copenhagen? Every season I spend a lot of time sourcing materials through new suppliers, and I always develop a strong relationship with my printer. None of my fabrics is from Denmark, but all the sample production and work with fur is done in Denmark, and some of the general production as well, though we are slowly trying to outsource this.

You decided to present your first show in Copenhagen. How come? It all happened very organically. I wanted to move back to Copenhagen for personal reasons, and then it

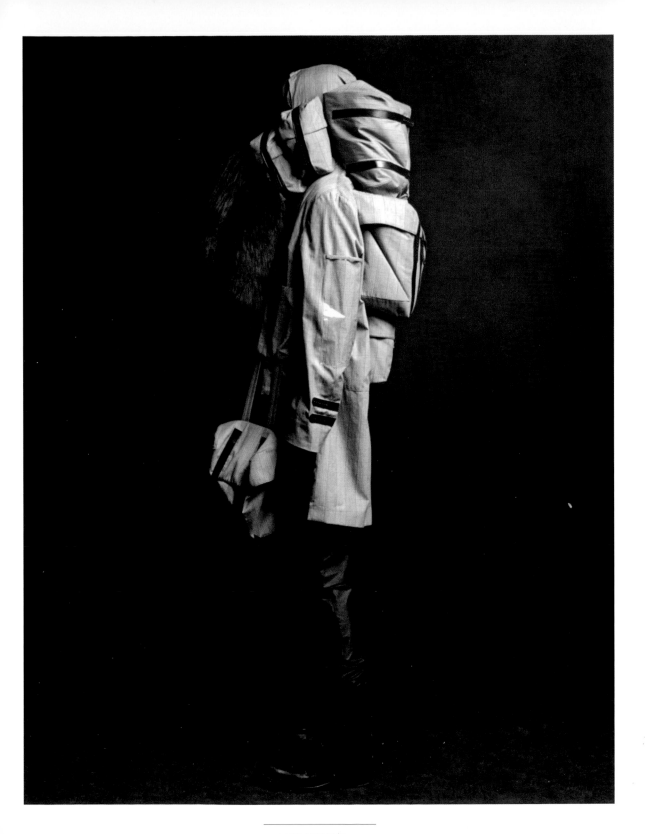

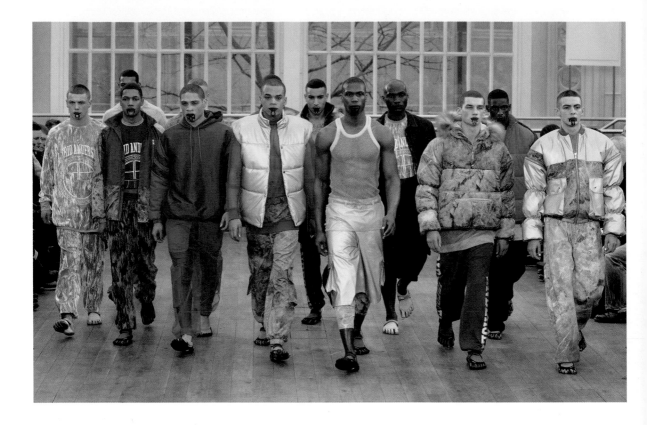

seemed somehow logical to launch the brand here. The dream was always to be part of the Fashion East 'MAN' show.

You did indeed present your collection as part of the acclaimed Fashion East show at London Fashion Week. How did you benefit from that experience? Fashion East has been the biggest support for my brand. They made sure all of the world's press and buyers would be aware of my collection. For a small designer, this is crucial. I'm so shocked when I look at how little talent support there is in Copenhagen. Being part of Fashion East's 'MAN' show was the biggest moment for my label so far – truly indescribable.

Tell me about your studio space. How do you work on a daily basis, and does your inspiration come from anything Scandinavian? I have a studio in the Nørrebro district, where I create all the sample production. For me the manufacture is such an important part of the design process that I hope always to keep this in my own studio. My inspiration comes from all aspects of life. Sometimes it's very personal and private, and other times it can be an obsession with a material or manufacturing detail. The only Scandinavian inspiration for me is the high quality of the manufacture.

What are you currently working on? I'm doing consultancy work alongside designing my collections. Every season is manically busy! I do technique development and creative consultancy for Kopenhagen Fur, and I just finished a design consultancy job for the Danish healthcare sector, which is something completely different to be involved in, and I am in contact with a massive sports brand. I also work as a visiting tutor at my old school, TEKO in Herning, which I love.

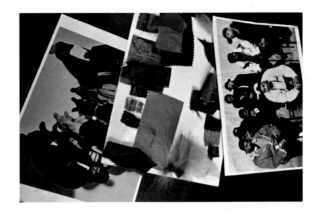

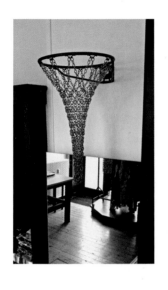

This page: Details of the studio space in Copenhagen.

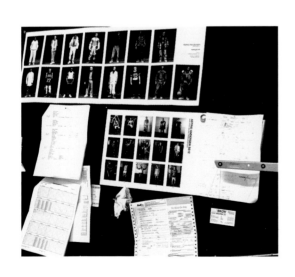

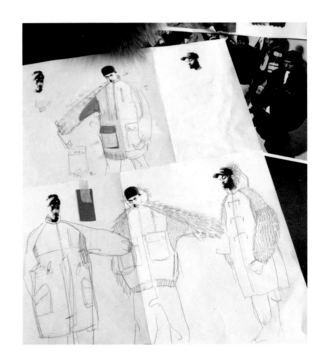

BEATE GODAGER

THIS NORWEGIAN DESIGNER, WITH A BACKGROUND AS A TAILOR,
HAS PRESENTED HER COLLECTION DURING COPENHAGEN FASHION WEEK.
SHE MOVES BETWEEN ART AND FASHION BY EXPERIMENTING WITH FABRICS WHILE STILL
CREATING WEARABLE CLOTHES. IN THE FUTURE SHE HOPES TO BE AT THE FOREFRONT
OF SUPPORTING ALTERNATIVE FORMS OF FASHION EDUCATION.

It is not that long since you graduated from Kolding School of Design. Tell me about your experience studying there. The school is very process-oriented and for me this was a good way to evolve creatively, finding methods for controlling my own artistic development. As for living in a small community, it's a bit of a challenge. Sometimes it's perfect to be surrounded by like-minded people and sometimes you need other influences. That said, I think the isolation made me focus 100% on my studies.

You are from Norway, but moved to Denmark. How come? Moving to Denmark was rather spontaneous. One week I decided that I needed a change of scenery, and two weeks later I was in Denmark with two suitcases and no place to live! I'd started considering applying to study fashion, and I knew that I needed to learn how to sew, then I found a tailoring school, so that's how I ended up here.

So you became a tailor… Tell me why you chose this road. I chose tailoring because I'd never sewn anything in my life, apart from what I'd learned in grammar school. I'd never really been interested in sewing, but I saw it as necessary for learning the technical side of making clothes so that I could execute my ideas in a proper manner.

When and why did you decide to form your own brand? My brand is in the early stages and I've just launched my first small collection. I would also like to contribute to improvements in the industry through a sustainable approach. I support the 'slow fashion trend', which is about durability and better quality, as well as smaller-scale production: quality before quantity. At the same time it's about respecting proper working conditions and the environment.

It must be quite hard to launch a brand now, but you persisted. Didn't you find any brand that matched your identity that you would have liked to work for? There are many wonderful fashion brands already that I'm sure would be very exciting to work for. To mention two companies I love: Martin Margiela (preferably before he left the company) and Comme des Garçons. But, as I mentioned before, my passion comes from being able to make the decisions myself. For me that is the core of my drive.

Do you have a team that helps you? Where are you based? I don't have a team, but I do have people who help – colleagues that I ask for advice, and friends who pitch in when it's urgent. I'm based in Copenhagen.

You say that you move between fashion and art. Can you explain that to me? Where is the borderline for you? The question of the borderline between art and design is a big discussion. A distinction between the two could be that design is a product that is usable. For me I think that a piece of clothing has an artistic value, even if it is a functional, usable product. However, if I could create whatever I wanted, without having to consider whether it's to be sold or not, my pieces would be much more experimental. I'm hoping I'll have the opportunity to do both in the future – showpieces and even art installations that don't necessarily have anything to do with clothes, as well as commercial pieces. For the time being, the more artistic side is reflected through details like playing with materials and small forms of deviation. For this collection, for example, I made coated fabric and put it in water and wrinkled it so that it kept the wrinkled shape when it dried. I also painted fabric to give it a stiff, rough look.

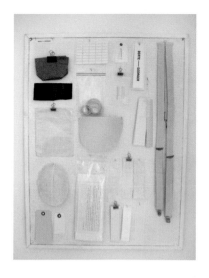

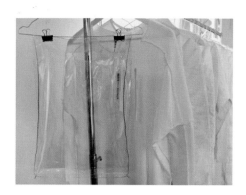

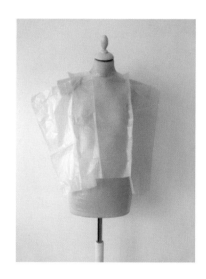

Above, right and below:
Details of the showroom and atelier in Copenhagen.

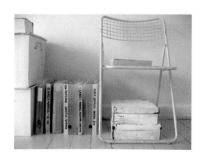

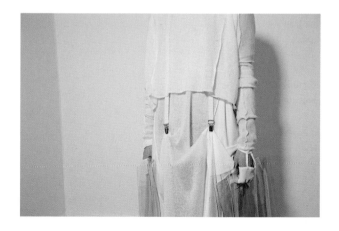

Do you sell your collection in any shops yet, or is it by personal order? At the moment I am in dialogue with several shops that are interested in my design, and some have already made orders, so that's great. I will also sell on some webshops. My graduate collection has been for sale at MUUSE since October 2011.

Where do you get your items produced, and how do you keep up with orders? I'm looking for production places at the moment, but this collection will be produced on a small scale so I might keep the production here in Denmark, depending on orders. I also do some customized pieces on request.

Tell me about where you will be and what you will be doing in the future. Hopefully I will be able to continue with my own brand and make a living out of it. In the long term, I'd like to combine my company with an educational model. I think that educating students can be a part of my company and other fashion companies since there are so many people working for free in this business. It's OK to intern for a short period during one's studies, but I would like to think that another educational model might be possible, which will enable students to stay longer with a company as an apprentice for a small salary. The student would get a more realistic view of the whole business, as well as a technical education, and the company would achieve a solid working relationship with a student instead of having to start from scratch by teaching new interns all the time. I believe that this model might also make it easier for students to get a job afterwards. It would be an additional form of fashion education; an alternative, if you like. I would also love to create or be part of a teaching programme for troubled teenagers. I'm hoping I can do that in the future.

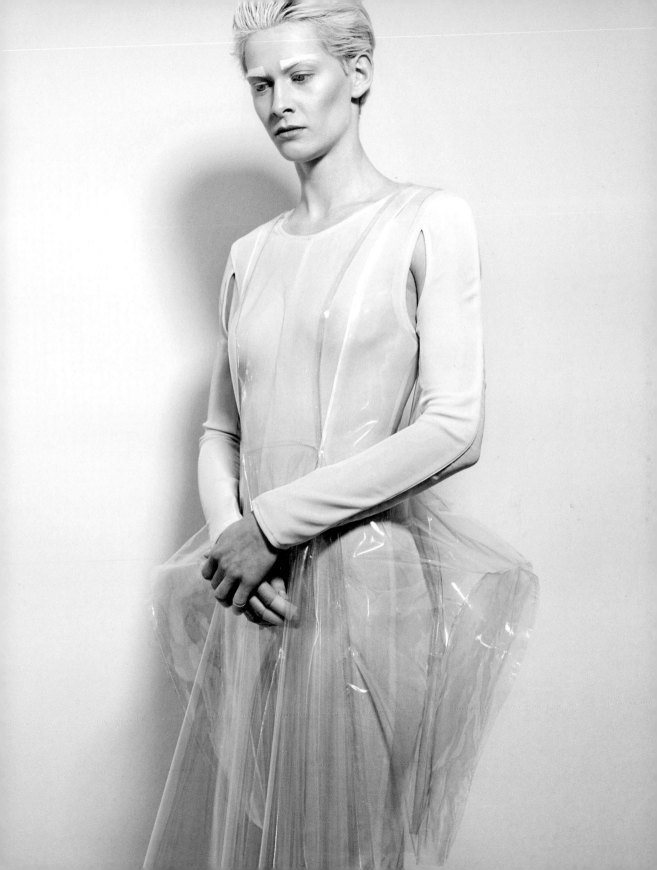

BRUUNS BAZAAR

BRUUNS BAZAAR WAS LAUNCHED IN 1994 BY TWO BROTHERS,
TEIS AND BJØRN BRUUN, AND QUICKLY BECAME ONE OF THE PIONEERS ON
THE SCANDINAVIAN FASHION SCENE. IT WAS THE FIRST BRAND TO PRESENT AN
IDENTIFIABLY SCANDINAVIAN YET INTERNATIONAL LOOK, AND, IN JANUARY 1999,
BECAME THE FIRST DANISH FASHION HOUSE TO ENTER THE OFFICIAL SHOW
CALENDAR IN PARIS. ITS CURRENT HEAD DESIGNER, REBEKKA BAY,
FORMERLY WORKED AS THE CREATIVE DIRECTOR AT COS.

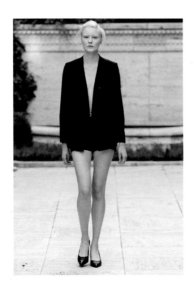

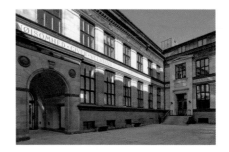

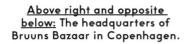

Above right and opposite below: The headquarters of Bruuns Bazaar in Copenhagen.

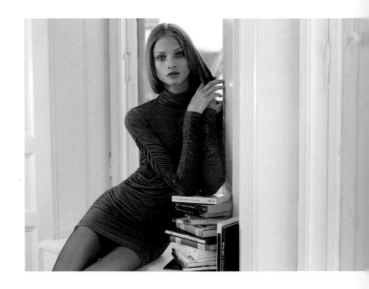

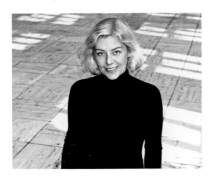

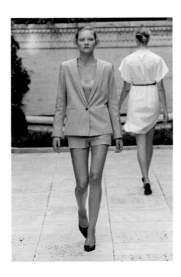

Above: Head designer Rebekka Bay.

Rebekka, tell me about your design background. You graduated from Kolding School of Design. What was that like? I graduated with a BA specializing in trend forecasting. At the time I was certain that I didn't want to design collections; I was far more interested in the inspiration process and the socio-cultural influences leading to the design than in the finished product. I really wanted to communicate ideas and concepts. Looking back, it might also have had something to do with my presentation anxiety. With so many talented designers around, I guess I was afraid of not measuring up.

I imagine you chose Kolding because you weren't from Copenhagen and your family lives in Jutland. If so, what were your aspirations, growing up there? I actually chose Kolding because it had a reputation for having more serious and more focused students than the Copenhagen-based design school. I don't think I was very specific with regard to my future or my aspirations. I grew up with a father who's a photographer but also employed at the Jorn Museum, which is a modern art museum in Denmark. I grew up with art, photography and museum visits as part of my daily life, and I've always gone to see art and discussed it with my father – not only the actual art on display, but also the presentation, the hanging, the buildings and architecture surrounding the art. I did consider architecture, journalism, even becoming a chef, and, well, I did have a go at art history…

Then you moved to London. What happened? Where did you start? I spent three years at Kolding and prior to that I'd spent a year at tailoring school in Aarhus, and some time before that I'd attended more industry-focused fashion courses. Design school didn't offer much with regard to trend forecasting and, after having spent four or five years constantly studying, I really felt like getting 'out there' to get some real experience. I moved to London with my boyfriend (now husband), with no contacts and no network. Someone put me in touch with the Danish trend forecaster Anne Lise Kjær. I started with her on a meagre salary but learned a lot within a very short time. After a year I approached Fitch, a big UK/US brand consultancy, and suggested they set up a London-based trend-forecast studio focusing on long-term trends and how to apply them. After a couple of years, with very long hours and a lot of travelling, I decided to become an independent trend forecaster and worked as a consultant for five years before I was approached by H&M to set up COS.

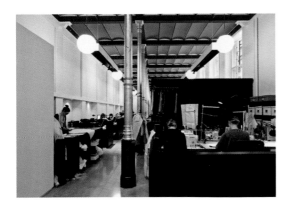

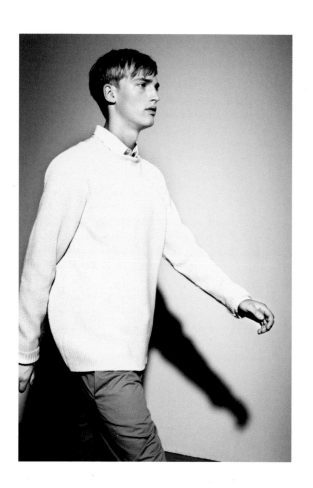

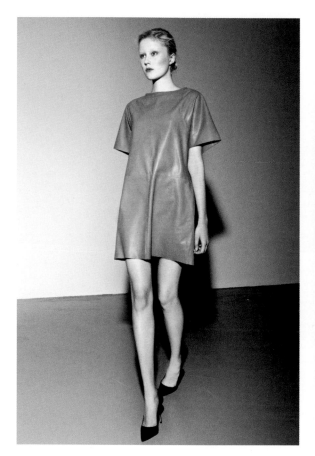

'Modern, understated
and crafted'

'I think what is really inspiring is when something that shouldn't really work together does'

You left the London headquarters of COS, the ultra minimalist brand, to focus on Bruuns Bazaar in Denmark. What do you plan to bring from the COS experience? Everything! Working at COS taught me the importance of intuition, common sense and focus. It also taught me the importance of good teamwork and strong individuals; the importance of balancing creativity with commercialism; the importance of testing and analyzing…

Tell me about your design process at Bruuns Bazaar and where the garments are produced. We start each season by getting together – all of us designers and design assistants – in a workshop, where we each present what we find inspiring. Out of that spring influences, themes and colours for the season, which are then translated into drapes, sketches and initial ideas. We are in constant dialogue – designers and buyers – and continually edit ideas and source new fabrics, finishes and trims. We also have in-house pattern makers and tailors, and that gives us the opportunity to try out ideas as we go. We then send drapes, drawings, technical specifications and requests to production, mostly in Poland, Turkey, China and India.

How would you describe the universe of Bruuns Bazaar that you are going to create? Modern, understated and crafted.

Where does your inspiration come from when you are designing a collection? Is it movies, books, music, travelling? I think inspiration can come from anywhere at any time in any form. I guess I'm often inspired by modernism in art, furniture or architecture, but an exhibition, a gallery space, a still life, a random colour harmony, a combination of materials can be equally inspiring. I think what is really inspiring is when something that shouldn't really work together does.

Bruuns Bazaar had quite a following in the 1990s. I can see how you are returning it to a modern state and applying a fresh cut. The silhouette is sharper, less ladylike. Is this the woman that you see on the street? That's who I am, and who I think is out there.

It seems as if the Swedish are particularly good at creating that crisp minimalism with these brands that have unique universes of shops, magazines, accessories, shows and events, and they do it so well that you really want to become the woman they represent. Why do you think that Danish fashion is so different? I think Danish fashion has always originated from a more bohemian fashion, which is funny considering our strong heritage in modernism and functionalism, but Danes are practical and comfortable. I think Danish design has a strong tradition of merging workmanship with design, and of considering products in relation to their surroundings. I'd love to address these aspects in the Bruuns Bazaar collections.

When you go out on the runway at the end of a show, are you already thinking about the next collection? What is going through your mind? Each collection always feeds ideas into the next. When presenting a collection, I'm always halfway into the next, and the one after that, and…

Where would you like to take Bruuns Bazaar? I would like for Bruuns Bazaar to be recognized as a modern fashion house with a strong Danish heritage and international appeal.

BY MALENE BIRGER

THE POWER WOMAN OF SCANDINAVIAN FASHION, MALENE BIRGER
DESIGNS, DRAWS AND IS MAD ABOUT PICASSO AND ART DOCUMENTARIES.
HER EMPIRE OF 950 SHOPS AND HUNDREDS OF MEMBERS OF STAFF AWAITS HER
EVERY MOVE. HER DESIGNS HAVE BEEN WORN BY THE DUCHESS OF CAMBRIDGE, SHE HAS
PUBLISHED AN INTERIORS BOOK ON HER HOMES IN MALLORCA AND DENMARK,
AND SHE PROVIDES WATER AND EDUCATION FOR THE CHILDREN
OF TOGO IN AFRICA. SHE IS UNSTOPPABLE.

How did you start out in fashion? Did you go to college, or straight to work? My interest in design began at an early age, inspired by my grandmother as well as by my mother's sharp eye for fashion. I sewed my clothes out of old fabrics and old clothes, and I dressed up in my grandmother's shoes, jewelry and lingerie, dancing up and down the road. We lived in a tiny village in the 1960s. It was not that normal! As a teenager I was very into fashion and did everything I could to create the latest looks – hair, shoes, make-up. *Saturday Night Fever* and *Grease* were my biggest inspiration. In 1989 I completed my degree in fashion design at the Danish Design School. I loved every single day of my four years there.

You have to be very determined and focused to get to where you are. I had a vision; I followed it and my ideas, while sticking to my 'universe'. That's it. A lot of work and a lot of passion. I don't do half-measures. When you work with the universe of By Malene Birger, everything is carefully thought through – first by me, then in close collaboration with my teams. Everything starts with design, and this runs through the rest of the company. Whether it's about a new collection, the show, the brand expression, a rib edge on a T-shirt or the graphics on our shopping bags, I'm a sucker for detail and I'm rarely satisfied and I think that everything we do should be done for a reason and have a story. Things are not just included for fun, unless the fun is serious.

You have created an amazing world, spanning brands, that still has a touch of Scandinavia, but do you get inspired on your travels? Yes, travelling is a great inspiration, but I like to travel in my mind, too. I love to work alone, to just be me in the creative process. I'm always on a journey, even if it's only in my own complex head! When I'm ready, I present to my creative teams. I don't feel Scandinavian or from any other nation. The brand is a definite result of the life I'm living.

Have you read a book called *The Allure of Chanel* by Paul Morand? Chanel's universe reminds me of yours, especially your beautiful office in Frederiksberg. Are there any people past or present who have inspired the universe you work in? Coco Chanel was a strong and clever woman. She did an amazing job nearly one hundred years ago. I haven't read that book, but I've read others about her. Her style is forever! I've been into black, beige and white for some fifteen years. I like to support my collections by surrounding them with natural colours in the décor and interior. I live like that myself. The collections mostly have colour and for me it gets too much, presenting colours in a room full of colours. Besides Coco Chanel, my hero is Mr Picasso. The man was unbelievably creative and versatile, and had an extreme work ethic. To me he is one of the greatest artists who ever lived. In general, I enjoy reading stories and watching documentaries about artists and historical figures – people who lived outside the box.

You decided to sell your shares, which must have been hard. How did you make up your mind? It was a radical decision to free myself creatively. I was drowning in daily business, staff and meetings; I wasn't very happy. It wasn't something that happened suddenly – it had been planned for a long time with my board and investors. They supported me.

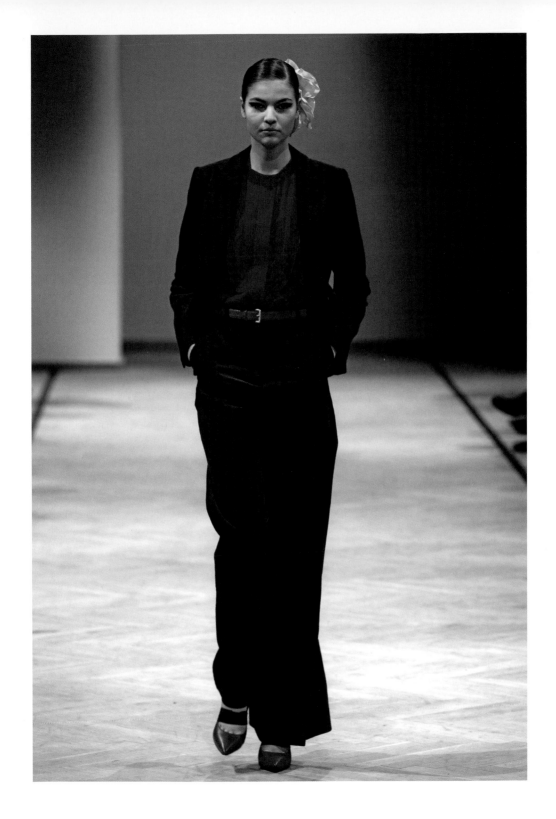

Below: The headquarters of
By Malene Birger in Copenhagen.

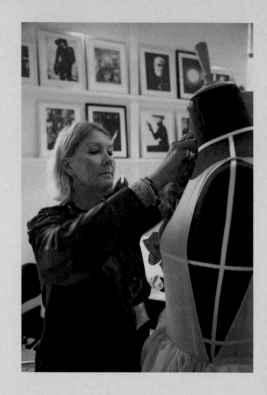

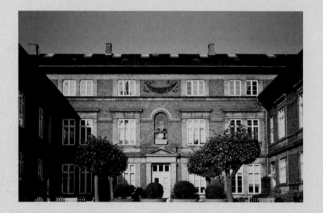

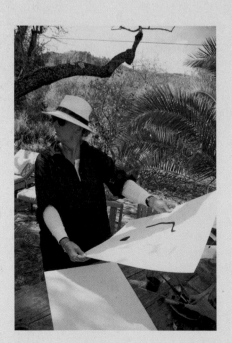

Above: Designer Malene Birger.

Below left: Malene Birger at
her home in Mallorca.

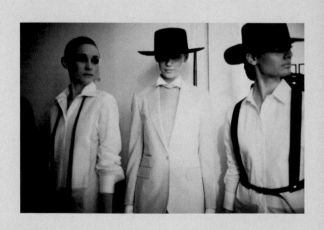

'I'm a sucker for detail, and I'm rarely satisfied, and I think that everything we do should be done for a reason and have a story'

ON SUCCESS

I'm still responsible for all the collections, all the creative developments and the 'universe'. I'm still the face of By Malene Birger. I'm the founder. But I've got time now to develop my other passions – art and interiors – and that's where I'm going to put my power in the future. It brings me so much joy, energy and new ideas for By Malene Birger. I need to develop to be able to develop the business. It's very simple, and it works!

I read somewhere that your business strategy is to keep things simple and to focus. How do you do that when you have your brand in more than 950 shops and 42 countries and have over 100 members of staff? Keeping focus and keeping it simple are essential. You have to make tough decisions in life, from resigning to breaking up partnerships, relationships, moving abroad or even selling your life's work. I definitely do not believe that success can be based on easy solutions and compromise. But I am quite shaken over how many people are terrified about making a radical change to their lives … so unfortunately there are many people who do not live the life they want. My work and the life I live and what I've said farewell to have definitely had their price. Keeping it simple is actually one of the hardest things to do in life. So the question should not be 'what do I do now?' but rather 'why do I do that?' Coming back to your second question, I'm a realist and I stick to my plan.

Are you still involved with UNICEF? Yes, I've been a UNICEF ambassador for eight years. In November 2011 I visited Togo, one of Africa's poorest countries. For many years By Malene Birger have worked together with UNICEF on providing the children of Togo with clean drinking water and education. It has absolutely been a life-changing experience.

Are there any magazines, books, films, anything else you can't live without? My Picasso books, my David Smith and Sonja Ferlov sculptures, *The Godfather*, my art movies, *Saturday Night Fever*; listening to Mozart's piano concertos and the jazz singer Jimmy Scott. Also my coffee in the morning and my imported rye bread from Copenhagen, since I live in Mallorca. And my husband, of course.

You seem to have so much positive energy. What advice would you give to a young person starting out today? The fashion world is the only creative business with no breaks, but with constant deadlines and new collections. Be prepared to give up a huge portion of your private life for many years. Believe in yourself, stay focused, follow your heart, don't compromise. You will mostly have to take all the responsibility, and be ready to take it: nobody will take it for you!

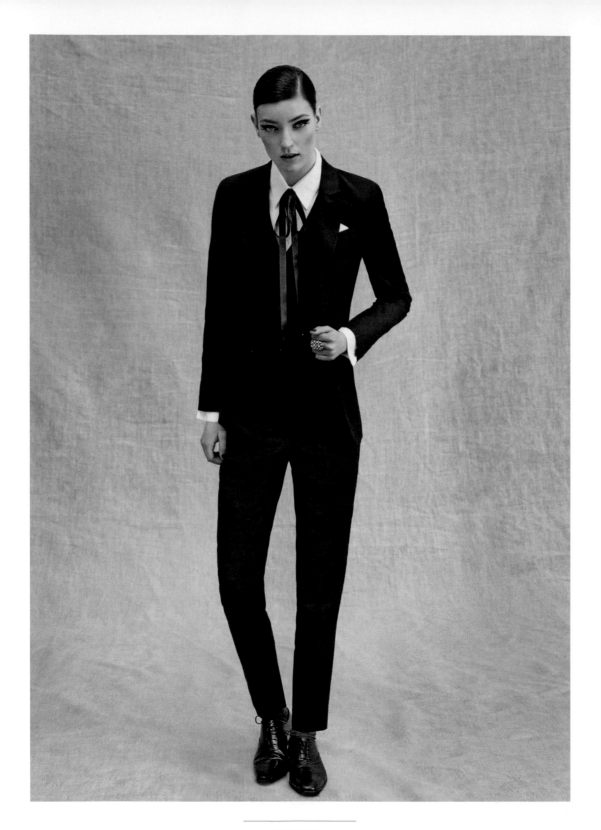

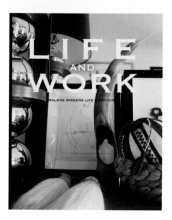

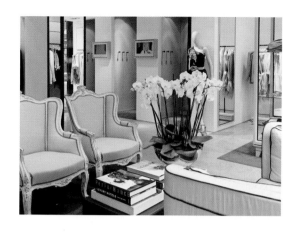

Below: By Malene Birger shop in London.

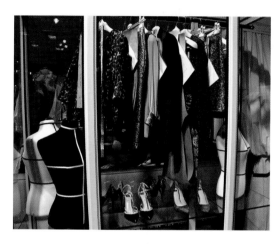

Above left and below left: Details from a book by Malene Birger.

Left: Showroom at the 'Gallery' fashion fair in Copenhagen.

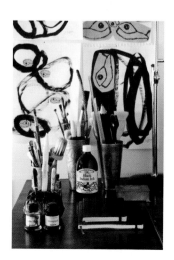

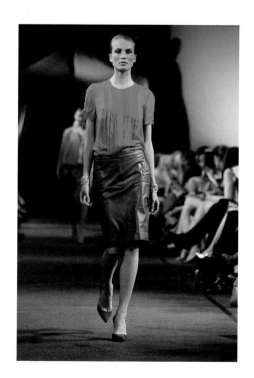

CAMILLA STÆRK

CAMILLA STÆRK IS AN INTERNATIONAL DESIGNER WITH A DANISH HERITAGE, WHO CAUGHT THE EYE OF HILARY ALEXANDER AT THE DAILY TELEGRAPH BEFORE SHE HAD EVEN GRADUATED. TODAY SHE LIVES IN NEW YORK, WHERE SHE MANAGES HER STUDIO WHILE ALSO WORKING ON FILM PROJECTS WITH HER HUSBAND, THE PHOTOGRAPHER BARNABY ROPER. SHE HAS HERSELF BEEN FEATURED IN A VOGUE ITALIA SHOOT, AS HER OWN PERSONAL STYLE IS IMPECCABLY BEAUTIFUL.

Tell me about your upbringing in Denmark. I grew up in the middle of nowhere. My life was spent on a farm with horses, dogs and cats; I was riding before I could walk. But my father's business is Danish furniture design, and I used to love going with him to his office in Copenhagen and experiencing a whole different world.

When did you decide that you wanted to work in fashion, and where did you study? As soon as I finished high school I went to Paris and Grenoble to study French for two semesters, then after that I went backpacking for a year around Asia, Australia and New Zealand. I then did my four years of study in London and graduated with a 1st Class Honours BA in Fashion with Textiles in 2000. When I started my studies, all I knew was that I had a passion for creating; a passion for art and design. During my third year I went to New York for my internship period and landed in the design studio of Patrick Robinson, Inc. That experience became a very important one. I met friends for life, and I was both encouraged and inspired to take the route of becoming a designer.

Your collection was presented at Browns in London. How did that help you to move forward? It helped immensely. The first person to take notice was Hilary Alexander. The day after my college graduate show *The Daily Telegraph* ran pictures and a story on the fact that my collection had been sold to Browns before I had even graduated. From that I was offered sponsorship to be one of the four designers for the very first Fashion East runway show, which was a huge success, with press and buyers attending from all over the world. So, two months after graduating, I was part of London Fashion Week, with a show and a sales stand, and that was the start of my business. It was surreal and amazing and nervewracking all at the same time.

Most of your designs are in black. Tell me about your relationship with the colour. It started with my own wardrobe from about the age of fifteen. What I love about only wearing black is the simplicity of it. I don't have to choose which colours to wear; instead textures, silhouette and the different shades of black become the focus. The subtle details become more important, and I like that. In my collections I like adding moments of colour and sometimes print, and again I feel that they become more important when shown in this sea of black.

You were also featured as yourself in a shoot in *Vogue Italia*. Who inspired you when it comes to style? My style has evolved slowly with time and with place, and I think most of all with the feeling of freedom to be myself.

You won Top Shop's New Generation Award three times. What do you think makes your design go straight to the hearts of buyers and the press? Individuality.

I read that you have developed a celebrity following. How did you nurture those relationships? Did the celebrities pick your collection from shops, or is it more friends along the way? A little bit of both.

What made you move from London to New York? Would you ever consider opening an office in Copenhagen? I fell completely and utterly in love with New York from the first encounter, so it was just a matter of timing. After ten years in London, and with a new business adventure ahead, the summer of 2006 felt like the right moment. Yes, I would absolutely love to open a space in Copenhagen as well in the future.

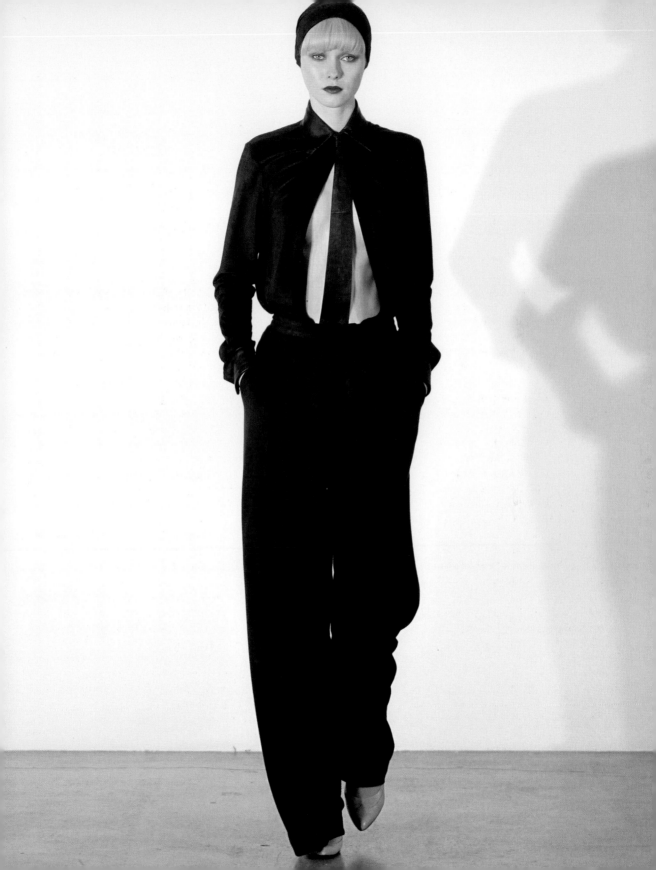

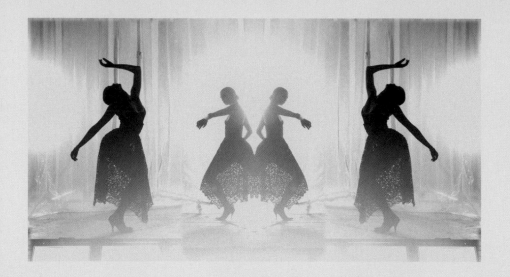

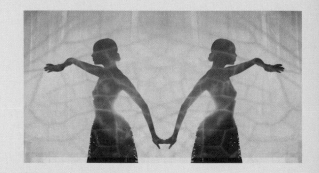

This page: Video stills of Royal Danish Ballet dancers by Barnaby Roper.

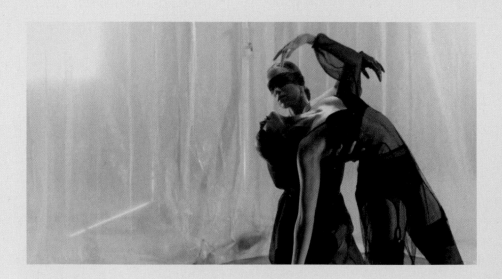

'When I started, all I knew was that I had a passion for creating; a passion for art and design'

ON FASHION STUDIES

You have worked on several collaborations, such as a bag and accessories line for Liberty of London and a men's fur collection for Kopenhagen Fur. Tell me about those relationships. Collaborations with a great variety of brands and companies are something I truly value, and I get to work within many different categories of design. It's inspiring, enjoyable and educational.

Tell me about the film you made with your husband Barnaby Roper, Sune Rose Wagner from The Raveonettes, and the Royal Ballet. We made the film *Vanitas* for the STÆRK SS12 collection, which was inspired by one of my favourite artists, Hans Henrik Lerfeldt. Sune and I had talked about collaborating for a while, and I had inspiring talks with Nikolaj Hübbe about the same thing, and suddenly everything came together in this one concept. Nikolaj cast the talented and beautiful Hilary Guswiler and Josephine Berggren of the Royal Ballet to be the performers in the film, and Sune composed this perfectly haunting soundtrack. We filmed one long day in a studio in New York, where Barnaby directed the set to his film concept and worked closely with the artists on the movements and the story. The film was shown on Nowness. com and screened at Tribeca Grand Hotel Cinema, New York, and at the Nils Stærk gallery, Copenhagen.

What are you working on at the moment, and where do you see yourself working in the next five years? I am working on the next steps for STÆRK. I see myself staying where I am and my work evolving into new territories. To be continued…

CARIN WESTER

SWEDISH DESIGNER CARIN WESTER WISHED FOR THE FREEDOM TO
BE CREATIVE. HER DREAM CAME TRUE, AND TODAY SHE MANAGES HER OWN BRAND,
AND HER COLLECTIONS CAN BE FOUND IN OVER 15 COUNTRIES WORLDWIDE. SHE ADVISES
THE NEXT GENERATION NOT TO BE AFRAID OF THE WORD 'MANAGEMENT'.

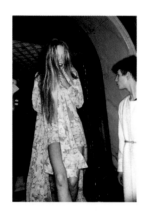

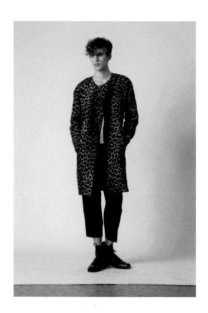

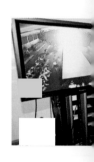

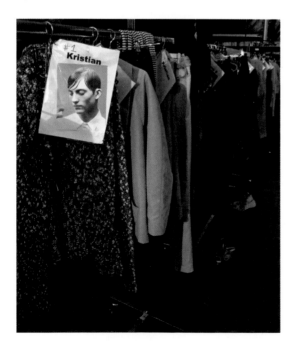

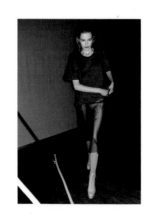

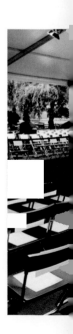

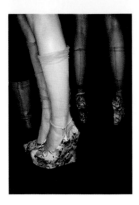

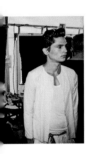

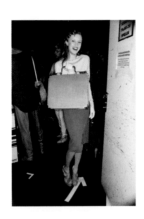

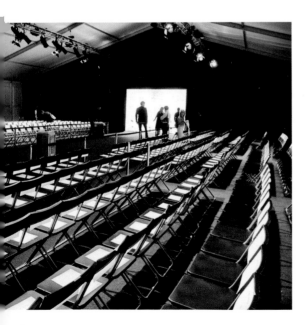

You have been working on your own brand since 2003, which is a long time, considering all the struggling designers around. What do you think has made your design last? There are most probably three different reasons why my design has lasted. The first is the fact that I didn't think so much about how to create a label but more about what was missing from the closet of a modern Scandinavian girl or boy. Secondly, I try to renew myself every season. I don't like the idea of repeating a successful style; I prefer to think that we can always bring something else. The third reason is to do with building up a team. Every designer needs to be surrounded by skilled people who help the brand to grow, organization-wise, production-wise and sales-wise.

Why did you want to launch your own brand back in 2003? After designing for a Swedish label [Paul & Friends], I was wishing for more freedom in my creativity. Then the idea of creating my own brand came along…

You graduated from Beckmans School of Design in Sweden in 1998. Do you follow what the new designers from the school are coming out with today, and can you see a change compared with the design back then? I always try to see the graduation show in May, since it's always so much creativity that makes you feel really happy.

Does your Swedish background translate into your designs? Or what is it that inspires you the most? It's difficult to say, since it can be so many things. Still I always come back to the core of my brand, which I call 'sharp poetry', where you can always find masculine cuts, playful prints and unisex pieces.

You were nominated as the Entrepreneur of the Year 2008 by Ernst & Young. How do you balance business with the creative side? It's always been a challenge to mix the two parts, ever since I started.

Where do you produce your collection? Is anything made in Sweden? The production is done in eight different countries and we keep a close relationship with the suppliers by visiting them as often as possible. The only things in the collection we still make in Sweden are the showpieces, which we produce in our studio. We produce in so many different countries due to each product requiring something different. It takes a lot of energy to put on a show, but at the same time it's all about attaining good quality at the right price. All our samples are made in Sweden; the patterns are created in-house and the graphics as well.

'I call the core of my brand "sharp poetry": you can always find masculine cuts, playful prints and unisex pieces'

ON DESIGN

There is so much great design coming out of Scandinavia. What do you think you all have in common? We share the same vision regarding how to dress. Nothing luxurious or snazzy; solid and compact collections, with wearable garments, at a price range that makes them affordable designed pieces.

If a new designer were to launch his or her brand tomorrow, what would your key advice be? To be very spontaneous with the design at first, then to put every effort into building the brand up, and to be unafraid of the terms 'management' and 'market'.

It feels as if you do a video every season as well. What is your opinion on fashion moving into the genre of film? I think that it's a very interesting move. It's always better to show a garment on a person in a live context. It brings an attitude. Still pictures can be extremely well produced, but there's an element of fakeness to them. Moving pictures are more real, in a way. Anything that brings inspiration around a collection is very important, such as the story about it, the music that matches, and so on.

Your collection is sold in more than fifteen countries all over the world. Did you play a vital role in creating sales, or do you have a dedicated team that takes care of that? From the start I had to care about that part of the process. Nowadays I have a sales team who are building up our network of retailers.

The look of your label is very recognizable. Who created the look? I'm the one who designs the complete collection, from the first drawing to the choice of colours and fabrics. Over time we've changed stylists and graphic designers, but I think their added value to my work has served the garments in the best possible way – not the reverse. That might also explain how we succeeded in creating the 'Carin Wester look'.

What are your plans for the future? Better, better and better … in all areas of our activity – design, production, sales, marketing. We can always improve ourselves. Somehow we have to stay a bit dissatisfied in order to transform that frustration into a positive energy to put down everything we did for the last six months and start from scratch for the upcoming collection.

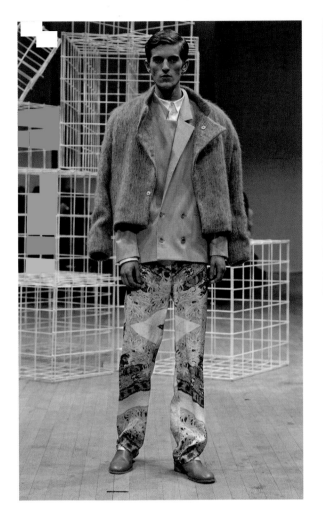
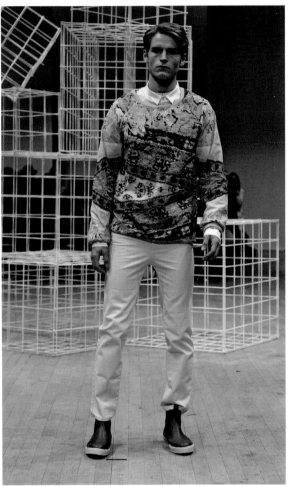

COS

ICONIC SWEDISH MINIMALISM IS PART OF THE DNA AT COS,
WHICH IS OWNED BY H&M BUT DESIGNED INDEPENDENTLY IN LONDON.
KARIN GUSTAFSON IS THE COS WOMENSWEAR DESIGNER, AND SHE SAYS SHE
DESIGNS 'FOR A GROUP OF FRIENDS'. IN ADDITION TO THE CONCEPT STORES
ALL OVER EUROPE, COS HAS RECENTLY OPENED SHOPS IN HONG KONG
AND KUWAIT … AND THAT IS JUST THE BEGINNING.

Karin, how did COS start out? COS came about as a business idea from the H&M Group, so there isn't a specific individual to be mentioned. The group was looking into new business developments, and we were lucky enough to identify what we believed was a gap in the market for a brand like COS.

Are you based with H&M in Stockholm? Our entire head office is based in London, but we've always considered COS to be an international brand with a Scandinavian heritage and feel.

Tell me about your own design background. Before relocating to London to study, I produced my own range in Stockholm. I joined COS in 2006, immediately after completing my studies at the Royal College of Art, and I became head of womenswear design in spring 2011.

Where does your inspiration come from? We look into a mixture of sources for inspiration – anything from art and architecture to new innovations in furniture design.

Who designs the shop spaces, which seem to take modern furniture and architecture as a reference? The original concept was created by the London architect William Russell. The stores have a modern look, with grey tones and subtle materials. These create a 'blank canvas' as a backdrop to the collection. We always try to create minimal, uncluttered, modern spaces, which are inspiring as well as easy to navigate.

Does H&M have any influence on your daily running of COS? We are proud to be a part of the H&M Group and we've only been able to achieve what we have so far because of the support that being part of the group offers. They support us daily on aspects such as logistics and IT, but in terms of design we are very much independent.

Tell me about who is in your mind when you design. I don't think of one particular woman, more of a group of friends that are strong-minded and appreciate minimal design and are slightly obsessed with clever solutions and functional details.

You have also launched a magazine and held events during the Frieze Art Fair. Even though the brand is available to everyone, you still have ambitions of being individual. Has this always been the DNA of COS? At COS we want to offer high-end design and high quality at an affordable price. We want to offer our customers the best product possible, but we also try to engage them within our shopping environments, from the music that we play in-store to our packaging and window displays, and even the COS magazine distributed in-store.

What are you currently working on. Are you expanding to any new countries? In 2012 we have so far confirmed we will open in six new markets, including our first stores outside of Europe, in Hong Kong and Kuwait. In-house we are all super-excited to see the reaction the brand gets further afield.

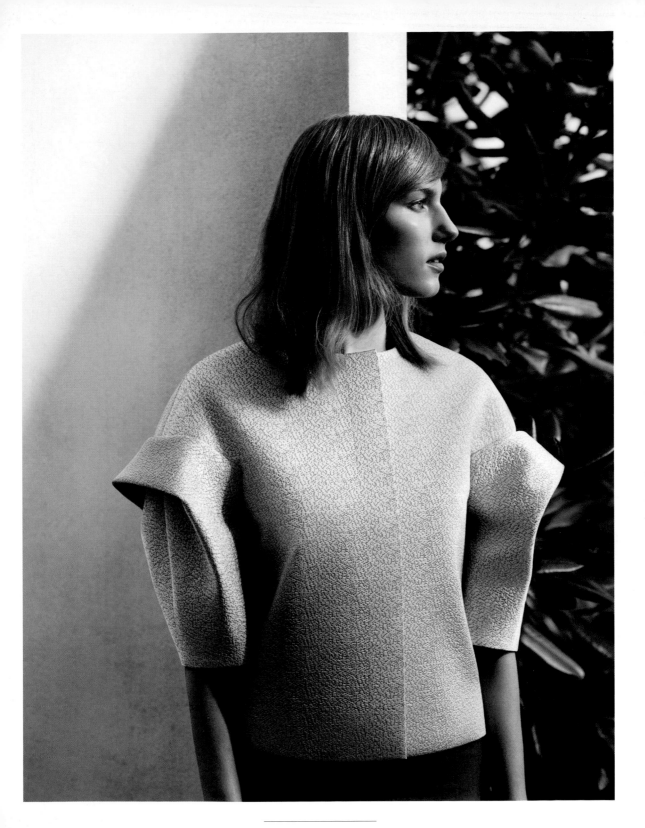

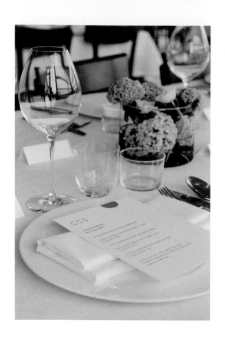

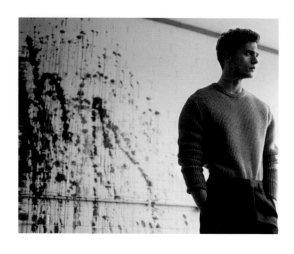

Left: Lunch served by COS during the Frieze Art Fair, London.

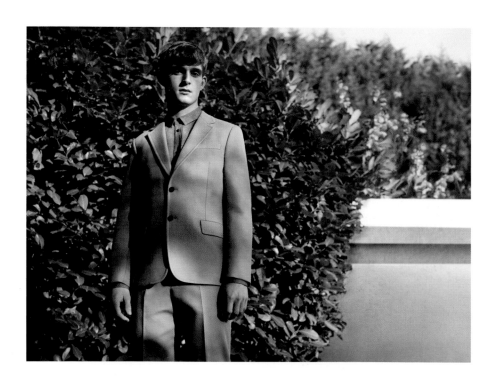

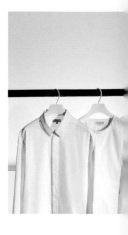

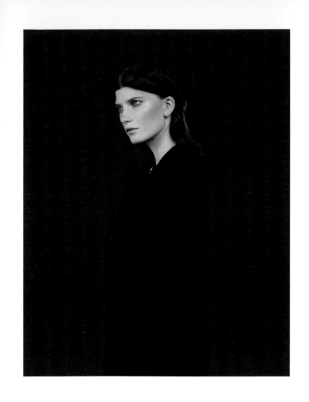

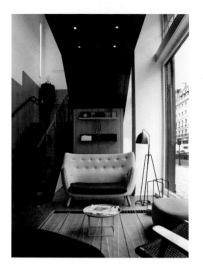

Above and below left: COS shop on Regent Street in London.

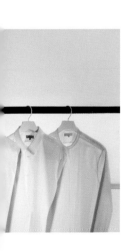

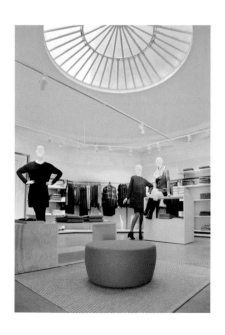

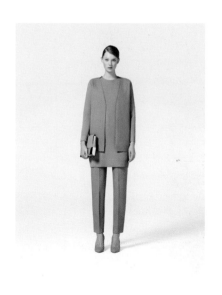

DAY BIRGER ET MIKKELSEN

FROM DANISH FISHING VILLAGE TO INTERNATIONAL MEGA-BRAND:
'DAY' CAN BE FOUND EVERYWHERE FROM HARVEY NICKS TO NET-A-PORTER,
AND IT JUST KEEPS EXPANDING. WITH FOUNDER KELD MIKKELSEN AT THE HELM
AND CONCEPT STORES FLOURISHING, THIS POWERFUL BRAND
IS NEVER AFRAID TO EXPERIMENT AND ADAPT.

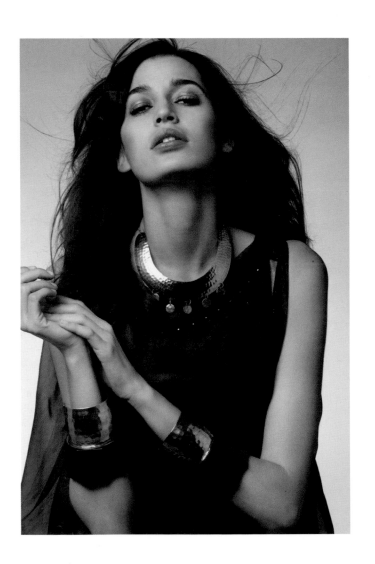

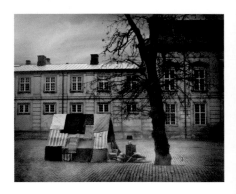

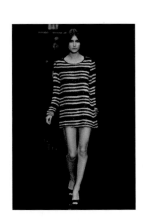

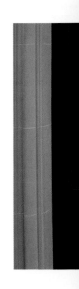

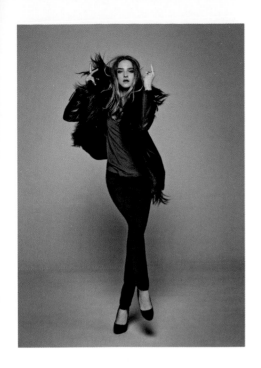

Keld, tell me about your upbringing. How did you start out in design? I grew up in the late 1960s in a small fishing village situated on the west coast of Denmark. I was introduced to 'the world of fashion' through a small shop selling Italian jeans, and that was a big eye-opener for me. It was love at first sight, and a love that has never stopped.

When and how did the idea of DAY Birger et Mikkelsen happen? After years of selling 'fashion' copies from Paris and London at attractive prices, I needed to make a mark for my own sake. I wanted to do original design. It was very much a process whereby I opened up the closet to see what was missing … and based on that I started my work.

Your clothing has been bought by many buyers, from Harvey Nichols in London to Galeries Lafayette in Paris. What makes your brand so successful? We put a lot of effort into making sure the brand is always worth looking at. We wouldn't have been successful if it wasn't for the fact that we feel passionately about what we do. The brand DNA of DAY has always been rooted in the contrast between the modern/classic look on the one hand and the ethnic look on the other. That has been our approach, and it seems to please people around the world.

Opposite right: DAY Birger et Mikkelsen Home campaign shot at the Christiansborg Palace in Copenhagen.

DAY is one of the few Scandinavian brands sold on Net-A-Porter. Did Nathalie Massenet approach you? How did it happen? I can't really remember how it happened exactly, but right from the beginning DAY was there, and we were and still are very proud to be one of the Net-A-Porter selected brands.

Your collections seem to be very influenced by travel – more so than most minimalistic Scandinavian brands. Does your inspiration ever come from being on a journey? I started my journey in India. I was eighteen years old and Calcutta blew my mind in a way that I will never forget. It's very natural for us to dig into the Indian culture and its beautiful people, both in terms of the way they actually look and in terms of their mindset. We love our Scandinavian heritage, but we need to add something to make it 'real'. If politicians could do the same, the world would look much better! Don't go crazy in your own bubble…

Is anything produced in Scandinavia, or is it mostly Asia? We produce in India, China, Turkey, Portugal, and Italy — again, a wonderful mix of culture and local craftsmanship.

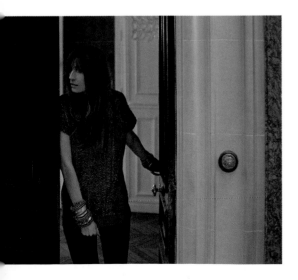

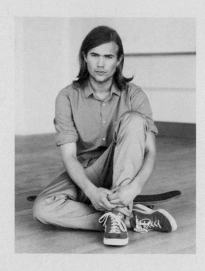

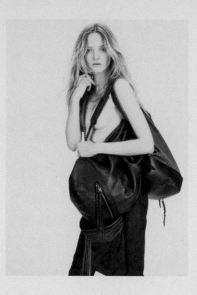

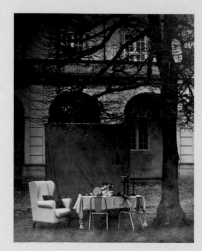

'We are and always have been on a journey of "intelligent evolution"'

———

ON CHANGE

'I opened up the closet to see what was missing ... and based on that I started my work'

———

ON INSPIRATION

'We wouldn't have been successful if it wasn't for the fact that we feel passionately about what we do'

———

ON DRIVE

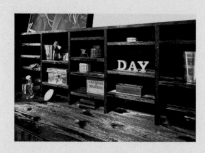

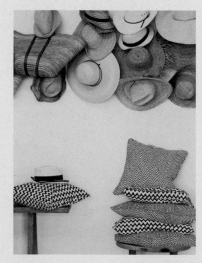

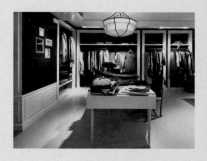

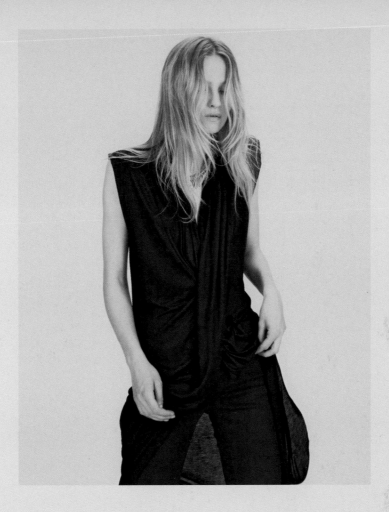

DAY is well known for its bohemian chic and the style has been copied over and over again. Now it feels as if times are changing and customers are not that romantic anymore. What is the next step for DAY? We are and always have been on a journey of 'intelligent evolution'. We picture the DAY woman as sexy and stylish; years back we thought of her as sensual and beautiful. I'm sure that this perception will be updated again in a couple of years. We don't want to force ourselves into a pattern that is not DAY. Even if fashion dictates it, we would always stay true to our beliefs.

So what are you currently working on? A DAY home/hotel perhaps? You know, it takes all we have to do DAY … and we do it 24–7. And it's great, I might add! We change our way a lot – a bit too much from time to time – but we never get bored. At the same time we're building a bigger retail department, and that is a lot of fun and a very hard road to travel, but let's hope we get rewarded some rainy day.

DESIGNERS REMIX

DANISH DESIGNER CHARLOTTE ESKILDSEN AND HER HUSBAND NIELS ARE BEHIND THIS SUCCESSFUL COMPANY, WHICH STARTED OUT USING LEFTOVER FABRICS. TODAY IT IS REPRESENTED IN MORE THAN 450 SHOPS ACROSS THE WORLD AND 15 CONCEPT STORES IN SCANDINAVIA. THE COMPANY PRODUCES SEVERAL COLLECTIONS, INCLUDING A CHILDREN'S LINE, AND ITS CLOTHING CAN BE SEEN ON CELEBRITIES AND ROYALS SUCH AS VANESSA PARADIS AND HRH CROWN PRINCESS MARY OF DENMARK. ITS HIGH FASHION COLLECTION IS PRESENTED AT LONDON FASHION WEEK.

Tell me about your upbringing. What made you choose design? I've always been very influenced by my parents and grandparents. My grandmother was a milliner and my grandfather made furniture. My father had his own company, where he worked as a creative director. Choosing design was very natural for me and I always had great support.

Where were you educated? I was educated in design management at Kolding School of Design.

Do you feel that Scandinavia has inspired your collections? I think it's important for me to express my heritage as a Dane, and I really appreciate where I come from. I'm very influenced by Danish architecture and, especially, Danish furniture. Designers Remix never went through the bohemian period and I'm not a very print-orientated designer, so I actually feel very in tune with the way architects think in terms of shape and silhouette rather than trends. I do most of my collections in black and Japanese cotton, wool or leather.

Tell me about the beginning of the brand. I was hired by IC Companys (where I met my husband) to start up new brands in 2002. One of them was Designers Remix. I made the first collection from 'leftovers' from the other brands, hence the name 'Designers Remix'. At the time it was very modern to customize clothes, and our collection soon became wanted by buyers all over. Then a time came when it just wasn't fun anymore and we realized we had to become more focused to take the brand forward. In 2006 this became a reality and I was able to make a more clear design DNA. Since then Designers Remix has been part of the official Copenhagen Fashion Week

show schedule and since 2010 the official London Fashion Week schedule as well.

Were you inspired by any past or present designers when setting up your house? Many! Arne Jacobsen, Hans J. Wegner, Verner Panton, Børge Mogensen – all Danish design heroes and all part of my heritage.

Your brand is now available in more than 450 shops across the world. How did you manage to develop this enormous success? I hope a big part of it is because people simply like the clothes I create, but I have to say that it also has to do with the business side. I have a great partner in my husband. He studied economics and has been great at choosing the right partners for us around the world.

I have seen your presentations in London. Is that an area you plan on continuing and expanding? I think it's a great challenge to play outside your home market if you want to push boundaries, and I was so excited about being approved for the official calendar so I took a chance. The future is hard to predict, and even more so today than it was just five years ago, but I definitely plan on expanding. For now the plan is to have more shops outside of Denmark.

Where are your collections produced? Is anything made locally? My collections and all of our prints are designed in Copenhagen at our head office. The production is done in Asia and Europe. Silk is great from China, denim from Italy, coated cotton from Japan. Corporate social responsibility is also becoming more and more important, and it's crucial for

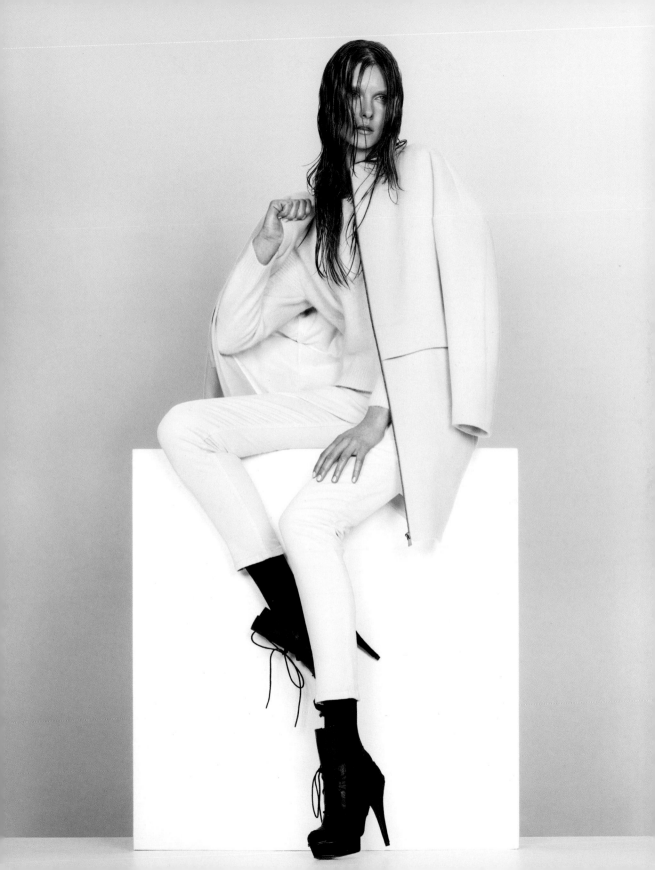

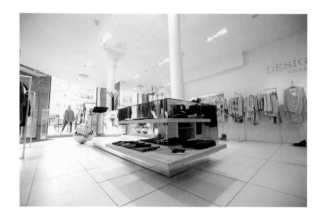

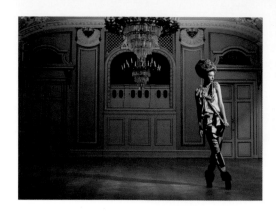

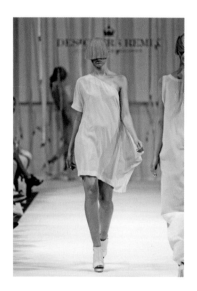

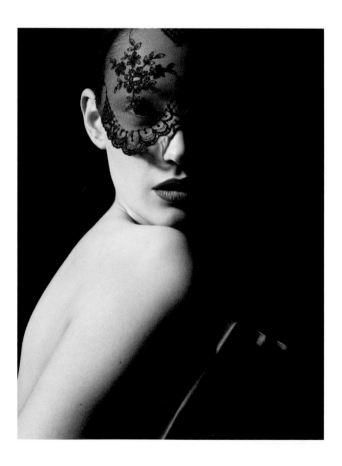

Top left: Designers Remix
shop in Copenhagen.

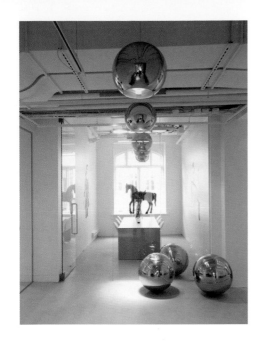

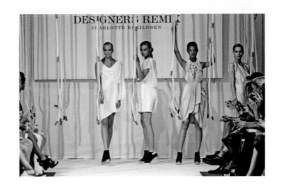

Left: A meeting room in the office above the Copenhagen shop.

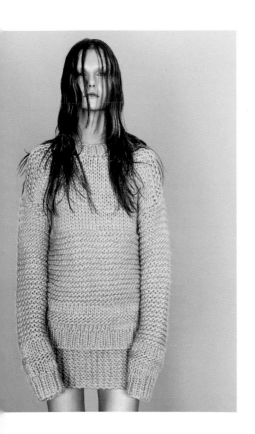

all my production that we put a high priority on adhering to the international standards set out by the UN and the International Labour Organization regarding human rights, employee rights, environmental protection and anti-corruption.

Do you have a muse when you design? Where does your brand's identity come from? I always work with the concept of 3D tailoring. I've been folding origami dresses and draping soft materials for many years. In other words, my muse is 'Japan meets Denmark'.

Hence your customized line of more avant-garde pieces… Who is your customer for these? The Designers Remix signature line is very much at the heart of my collections. This line is targeted towards the international market. I often feel inspired by the culture I live in, be it movies, art or cities.

Is IC Companys still involved in the process? Designers Remix is half owned by me and my husband and half owned by IC Companys. They owned the company outright in the beginning, but later my husband and I were able to buy half.

What are you planning for the future of Designers Remix? Right now my plan is to stay focused. Europe is going through a rough time and I feel as if controlling the values and sticking to the concept are musts rather than risky investments. I believe in creativity, and the future is all about making wonderful collections and having a lot of fun!

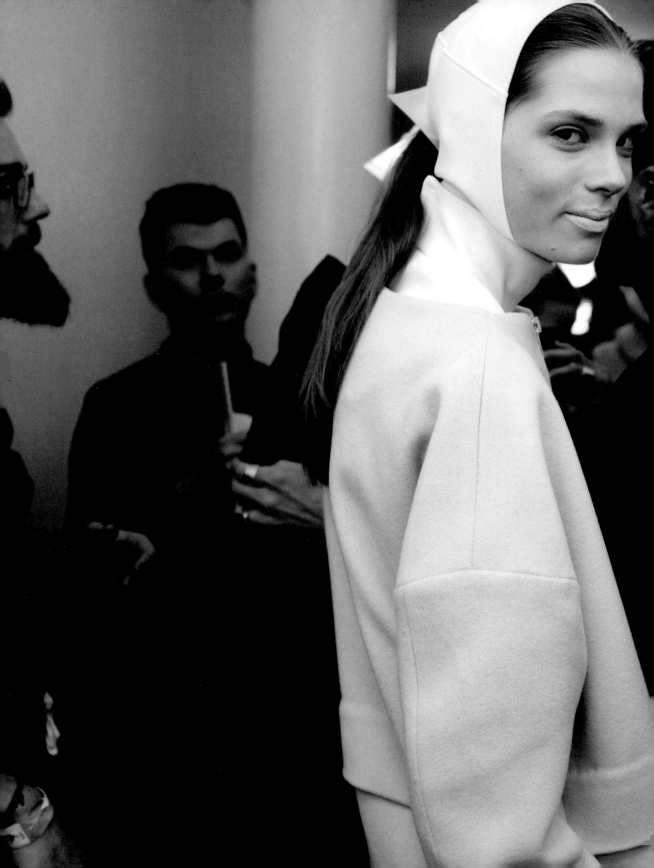

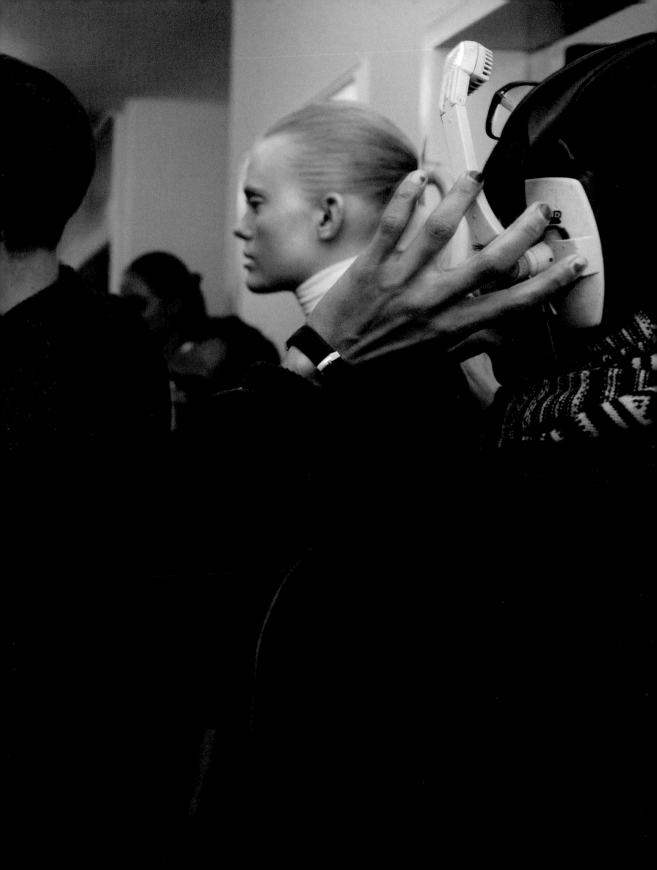

EYGLO

IN 2006, AFTER GRADUATING FROM THE ICELAND ACADEMY OF THE
ARTS AND INTERNING WITH BERNHARD WILLHELM, ASFOUR AND JEREMY SCOTT,
EYGLÓ MARGRÉT LÁRUSDÓTTIR STARTED HER OWN LABEL, FOR WHICH SHE LOVES TO
EXPERIMENT WITH PATTERN CUTTING AND TAILORING. WITH NINE OTHER DESIGNERS,
SHE ALSO CO-OWNS KIOSK, A SHOP ON LAUGAVEGUR IN REYKJAVIK.

Can you tell me a bit about your background? I was born in 1981 and grew up just outside Reykjavik. I was never an artistic kid and couldn't care less about clothes. Instead I was obsessed with Lego. I was really into the structure of buildings and loved going to visit people to see how their houses were planned. I always thought I'd be an architect... As a teenager I went to a business-related school, but I changed overnight. I started making my own clothes around the age of seventeen because I couldn't find anything interesting enough here in Reykjavik. There wasn't much to choose from at the time. That has changed dramatically. But there was no turning back after I got into fashion. Now I can't imagine doing anything else.

When you were seventeen, making your own clothes, was there a scene in Reykjavik? Did you feel as if you belonged to something? No, there was no scene – not that I noticed, at least. I guess I looked quite ridiculous!

What was the Iceland Academy of the Arts like? It was quite new. I graduated in 2005 and I think that was the second year of fashion graduates there. We had a lot of teachers from abroad, and Linda [Björk Árnadóttir, head of the fashion department] helped us get internships, which was really good. Finding fabrics was a bit difficult, though. That bothered me the most. It's so expensive just to get the basic fabrics here. Instead you have to try to be inventive – screenprinting, etc.

Where does your inspiration come from? I usually know the next theme months before I start working on a line. Once I had to take my son to the hospital and my eye was caught by an X-ray of a hand on the wall. That was the beginning of my AW11 collection. Then my son came home from the library with a dinosaur book, and SS12 came along. Now I'm working around crop circles after watching the TV series *Ancient Aliens*. For the next winter collection I'm thinking about looking to Icelandic nature for inspiration...

You interned for Bernhard Willhelm and Jeremy Scott, among others. How come? Your design isn't as crazy as theirs. You seem to have more focus on the pattern cutting and structure. I was very into the crazy stuff as a student. But I needed to find balance after graduation, and my first line was a really classic one. Now I'm trying to push myself a little bit more by using unusual (ugly) fabrics with really beautiful ones. I love my job!

Iceland is a really special place, but very isolated. How do you keep track of the world outside? It's tricky. It's good to be able to travel a lot, meet new people and be active socially when I get the chance, but it's also good to have some peace in which to grow ideas. There's so much space to think, and hopefully make something special.

Do you see yourself as an Icelandic brand? I don't think I'm a typical Icelandic designer, but of course I'm immune to seeing that in myself. You might just recognize it because I'll probably have winter swimsuits. We're always swimming here because we have a lot of hot water, and it's hard to get nice swimsuits, I think. I can give you one with pleats and zippers in the back. It will come in dinosaur print and black.

Yes, please! Do you think what you do is more of a job or a lifestyle? Definitely a lifestyle. I'm at my happiest when I'm working. In the future I just want to keep on pushing myself into trying new things ... and to be sold in more stores around the world, of course.

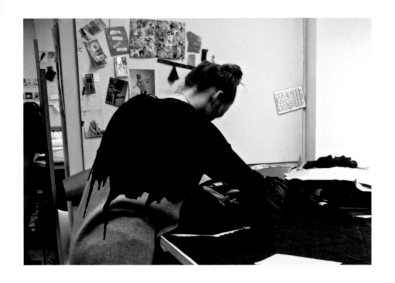

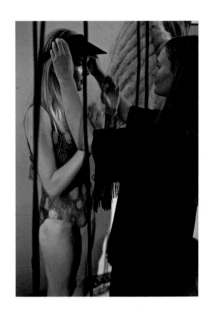

Above: Designer Eygló in her workspace in Iceland.

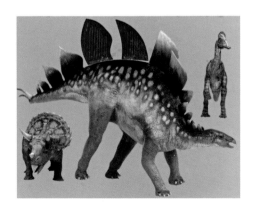

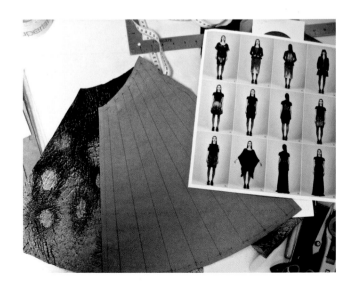

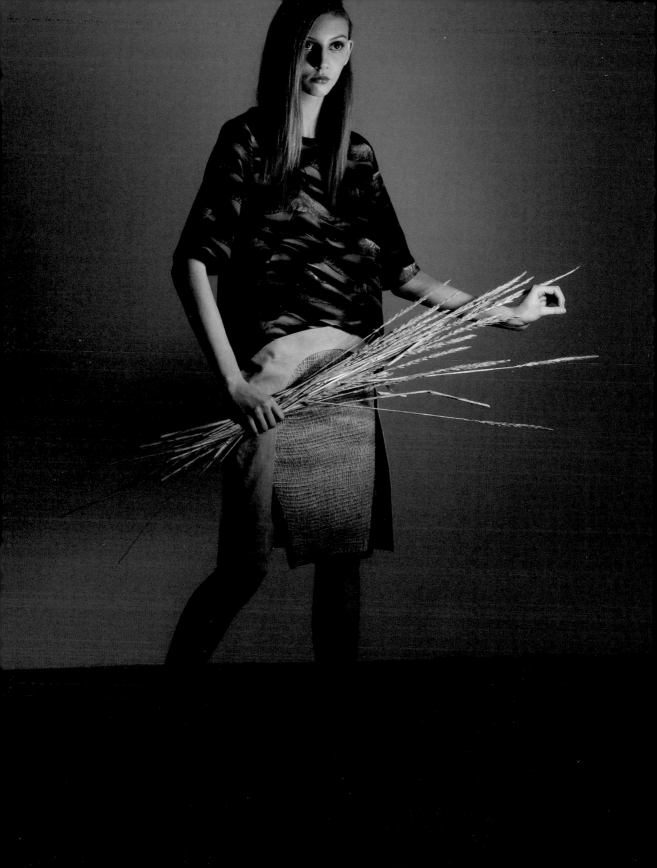

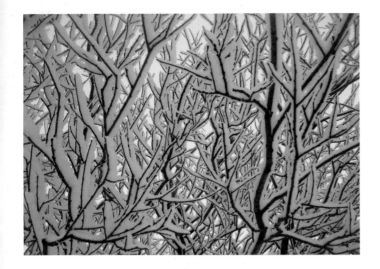

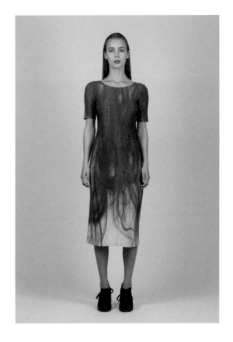

Left: Icelandic landscape inspiration for the AW12 collection.

Left: Eygló.

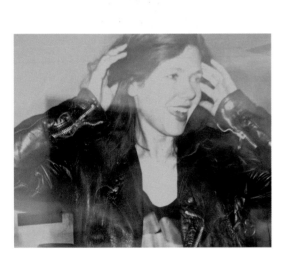

'I'm trying to push myself a little bit more by using unusual fabrics with really beautiful ones'

V AVE SHOE REPAIR

THE DUO ASTRID OLSSON FROM SWEDEN AND UK-BORN LEE COTTER STARTED THEIR BRAND IN 2004, AFTER MEETING IN STOCKHOLM. TODAY THEY HAVE STORES IN SWEDEN AND SINGAPORE, FAMOUS CLIENTS, A STUDIO IN A BEAUTIFUL OLD BREWERY AND A DREAM OF TAKING THE NEXT STEP FORWARD – POSSIBLY A SHOW IN PARIS.

Tell me about your upbringing in Sweden. Lee and I have quite different backgrounds. Lee is half-English and lived in London until he was eight. Then he moved to the north of Sweden, until he finally went to Stockholm as a teenager. I was brought up in a suburb in Stockholm and moved into the city in my teens. I believe that we have one very important thing in common: we thought that we could do what we believed in as long as we worked hard. Honesty, hard work, passion and creativity are probably what make us so much alike.

What is behind the name 'Fifth Avenue Shoe Repair'? V Ave Shoe Repair is, in short, a dedication to craftsmanship and the love of fabric and working with your hands. The name was inspired by a small shoemaker's in London, which takes in old, worn-out, handmade shoes and restores them and sells them again. This, for us, is pure love.

You are very experimental with fabrics. Where does this touch come from? I think it's just our love of fabrics, tailoring and manufacturing. We keep collecting little swatches of things wherever we go. Not just textiles; almost anything could be a garment, right?

Yes, anything! But how do you balance experimentation and creativity with the more commercial side? Today I believe this balance is more important than ever. The secret is to find small inventions and creative solutions in details, stitches and cutting that give the same feeling of flow, whether you're making a commercial garment or creating a bigger silhouette.

Do you sell your showpieces to any secret clients? Yes, we have both very famous artists and some regular customers who like to appear in really spectacular things, including for weddings, but we prefer to keep that to ourselves.

You have two stores in Stockholm and one in Singapore. Are you going to branch out to other countries soon? Our vision is to have one store in each of our favourite cities, such as Paris, Hong Kong, Tokyo and Berlin. But for now we are more focused on working with our existing stores and our online shop.

Tell me about your design process. Do you start with a sketch or drape? How does it develop? Our design process is always a stressful and sometimes even painful process, which we for some reason cannot live without. I would say we start with both draping and sketching at the same time, so as to let them rub off on each other. The most inspiring things are sometimes the things that just happen … maybe by mistake. Designing is a lot about allowing yourself to wait, to have patience, and then to work fast.

Your design studio is situated in an old brewery dating from 1840. Tell me about the atmosphere there. We are very fortunate to have this great space to work in, with lots of open areas and white floors and walls. We've kept the old brewery features, for instance a floor sloping towards a tap in the floor of the hall. The building has had a long life, and, since it's an industrial building, we don't need to be that careful here. In a studio it's necessary to be able to splash colour on the floor, and use a hammer and saw as well as heavy sewing machines.

How do you feel you have developed from the start to now? Have you changed your approach in design? Does the business side take over sometimes? Since it

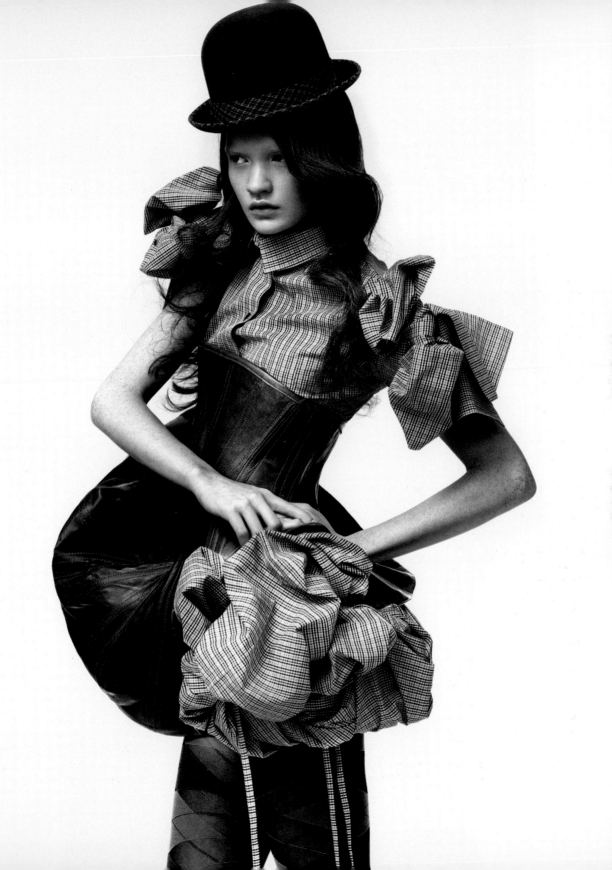

'The secret is to find small
inventions and creative
solutions in details,
stitches and cutting'

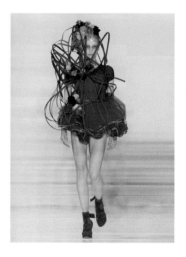

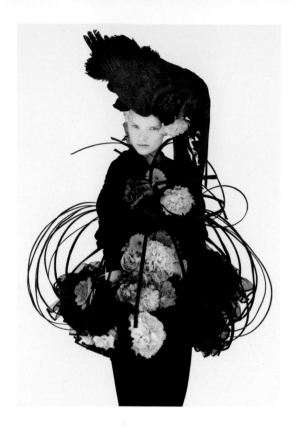

started as just a small project of fifteen garments, I think we've come very far. Over the years the approach has changed. It has to, since you always try your best to become a better designer, a better boss and a better manager. I would say we've lost a bit of the naivety that we started off with. But we've also gained a lot of knowledge, met a lot of fantastic and inspiring people, and learned that things have a way of sorting themselves out. And, yes, it's not only about making beautiful garments. The business side of running a company is sometimes the biggest part. So you have to really love what you do to work in fashion.

Where do you source your fabrics? Is anything made in Sweden? We source fabrics at the Première Vision in Paris, which is the biggest fabric fair, held twice a year. We buy a lot of Italian fabrics, which are always beautiful quality. We also always look for fabrics that are produced locally to where we manufacture the garments – in Portugal, Italy and Turkey.

We strongly believe that it's better to buy a local fabric and cut out the long transportation to save the environment. In Sweden it's a bit difficult to find high-level production, but we have in the past done a bag collaboration with Alstermo Bruk, a traditional Swedish bag manufacturer founded in 1804.

Are you planning on continuing to showcase your collection in Stockholm? You have also presented it in Copenhagen. Will you return there, or will you go somewhere abroad? As you know, we love doing shows! We love the feeling backstage just before the opening and the possibility of making our vision come alive, if only for fifteen minutes. Paris is the capital of fashion and we will always be present in showrooms for the Paris weeks, but since we are based in Stockholm our shows and presentations will most likely be held here for now – especially in the spring and summer, when Stockholm is a fantastically beautiful city.

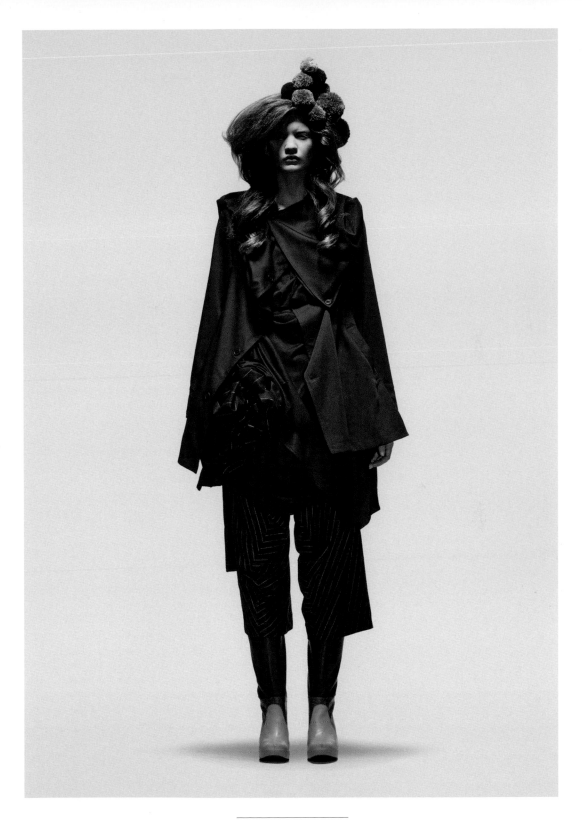

FILIPPA K

THE SWEDISH DESIGNER FILIPPA KNUTSSON NEEDED MORE FUNCTIONAL GARMENTS IN HER WARDROBE. THIS WAS THE BEGINNING OF THE MINIMALISTIC BUT EASY-TO-WEAR SUPER-BRAND, FILIPPA K, WITH STORES ACROSS THE WORLD. TODAY FILIPPA IS A GLOBETROTTER WHO FITS A PILATES SESSION OR TWO INTO HER BUSY SCHEDULE. KEY MEMBERS OF HER STAFF ARE MARKETING DIRECTOR EVA BODING AND HEAD OF DESIGN NINA BOGSTEDT.

Eva, why did Filippa K start out with her own brand? Filippa Knutsson felt a need for simple functional garments with a clean design – essential pieces to build a wardrobe around, easy to combine and long-lasting in both style and quality. That was the start of Filippa K in 1993 and is still the essence of the brand today.

Did Filippa start by herself, or did she have partners? She started Filippa K together with her husband at the time, Patrik Kihlborg.

How did it become so successful? What was the key? The brand fills a clear need. From the start it matched long-lasting style with high quality. It attracts many people thanks to a wearable and comfortable product with an effortless design.

You sell your collections in more than twenty countries. When did the expansion really start to take off? Actually from the start. First we met with big success in Sweden, Norway and Denmark. Over the years the strongest markets have been in northern Europe, but we have loyal Filippa K customers in all kinds of countries, from Australia to Russia.

Is Filippa Knutsson still the main designer? How is the company managed today? Nina Bogstedt, who has been with the company for almost fifteen years, is the head of design. Filippa Knutsson doesn't work within the company on a daily basis, but she is still one of the biggest owners, a member of the board and a big inspiration to the company.

You always have great campaigns, with models like Alana Zimmer. What is the idea behind these? Our campaign has the important purpose of connecting with and moving our customers, making them feel the brand's personality.

Do you produce anything in your collections locally in Scandinavia, or is everything from abroad? Special design projects are produced in Stockholm, but apart from that we have 60% of our production in Europe and 40% in China.

Is the head office located in Stockholm? Yes, but we work closely together with local Filippa K organizations.

Nina, when you begin to design a new collection, do you start out by working on the previous one? What is your work process like? Every Filippa K collection has a core of essential pieces that stay the same over the seasons: only small changes are made to make sure they stay up to date. The rest of the collection evolves around the core. We aim to fill the everyday dressing needs of our customers and ourselves, and we have a clear purpose for every piece.

Who decides where to locate the shop-in-shops? They all seem to be in beautiful buildings. Our local business owners are responsible for the expansion through brand stores and shop-in-shops. The central organization delivers a store concept for these new locations. So it's a combination of local knowledge and central expertise in what is best for Filippa K stores.

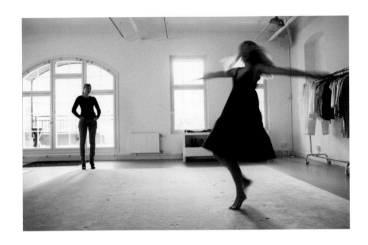

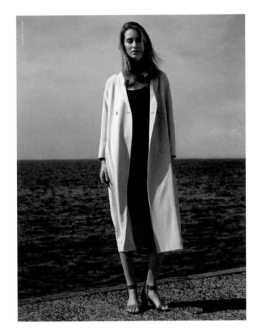

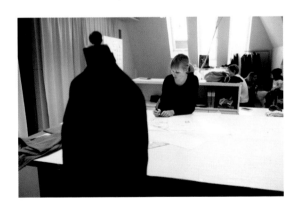

Above left: Filippa Knutsson (left) in the showroom at the head office in Stockholm.

Below: The Filippa K atelier.

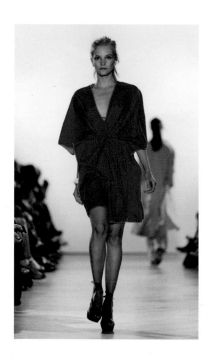

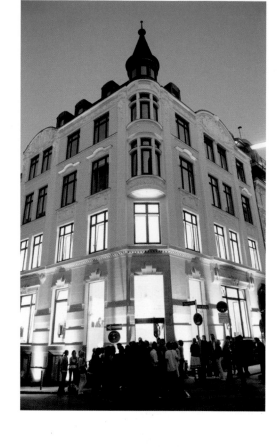

Right: A Filippa K
shop opening in Hamburg.

Below: A presentation in Oslo.

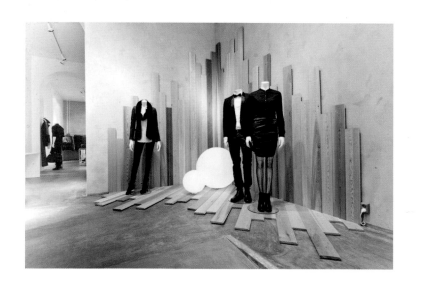

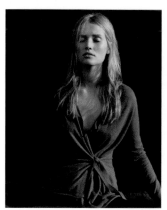

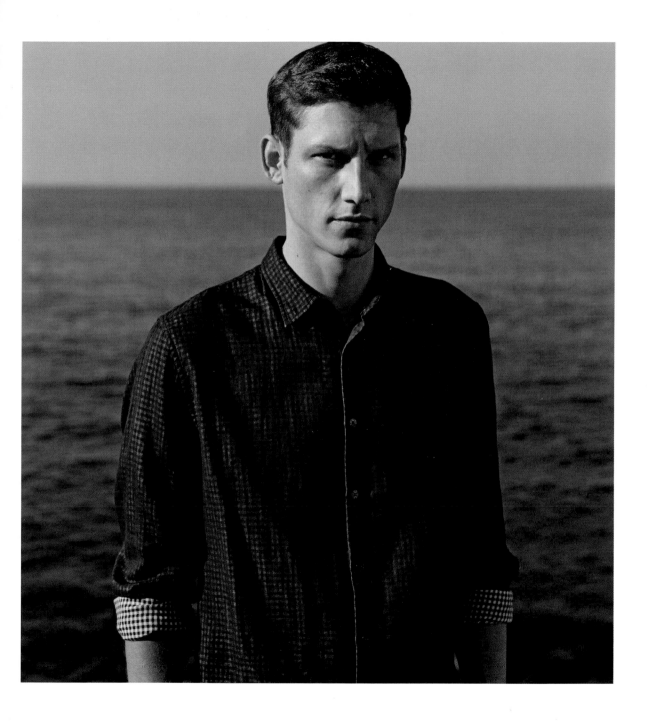

GAIA

COLOURFUL BUT ETHEREAL COMBINATIONS ARE INCORPORATED
WITHIN GAIA'S AESTHETICS, ALONGSIDE INSPIRATION TAKEN FROM THE
RUSSIAN AVANT-GARDE. GAIA BRANDT GRADUATED FROM CENTRAL SAINT MARTINS,
BUT HER CURRENT BASE IS IN COPENHAGEN, WHERE SHE INTENDS TO
DEVELOP ONE OF DENMARK'S FRESHEST KNITWEAR BRANDS.

Gaia, your name is very beautiful and special. Where does it come from? It's connected to ancient Greek culture, where it was used as a term for Mother Earth. My rather untraditional childhood was spent alongside alternative and creative parents, who manage an organic garden, something they've been doing since the 1970s. So my name fits my background, philosophy and brand identity rather well.

You founded your brand in 2009 in Copenhagen, but studied in London at Central Saint Martins. Tell me about that experience. The coursework was very independent, in a creative and encouraging environment. In many ways it was a great and educative stay for me in London. At times, I must admit I miss the possibilities, perspective and energy of that buzzing city. Nonetheless those elements also inspired my return to quaint Copenhagen to further develop my brand. As a very driven person, I aimed to work independently, following my own choices, which of course at times has been challenging.

What did you study at Central Saint Martins? I studied Fashion Design with Knitwear, which allowed me to focus on knit techniques, fusion of original materials and quality construction – central in my designs.

When you combine vintage fabrics with your knitwear, I presume that the collection has to be more limited. Are the fabrics from Scandinavia? All my materials are lush and exclusive, always carefully selected after a long research process. They might be vintage fabrics or materials that are traditionally used for furniture or curtains, or they might come from dead stock and be treated or altered by me. I think sustainability is an important theme for future consumption. I like to contribute to a better world, in my own way, by re-using parts of vintage materials and focusing on responsible production processes.

You combine the precise cut of a tailor with knitwear that is more chunky and, I guess, complicated or time-consuming to produce. Where do you manufacture your garments? The collections all consist of garments handmade here and quality production in Europe. I previously trained as a tailor and have a great passion for craftsmanship, so I aim to make the more challenging pieces in my own studio, which is indeed time-consuming but very much worthwhile.

Are you inspired by Scandinavian aesthetics? Usually I look more towards the Russian avant-garde and graphic German artists and personalities from the 1920s and '30s for inspiration. I like to dabble in colours and graphics from Dadaism and Surrealism. I gain a lot of inspiration from the materials I use, where the extensive process of construction is very rewarding.

Do you present your collection abroad at any fairs? GAIA is growing organically and calmly, so we are exploring the market. For the next few seasons the focus is on Scandinavia, the UK, Benelux and Germany, also with strong interest from Japan and the Asian market. We aim to gain more exposure and sales points over the coming seasons.

The inspiration you have on your mood board is very much about storytelling and the old, rather romantic times of innocence and style. How do you feel you transfer these to your designs? For me it has always been interesting to research old photographs from books, antique

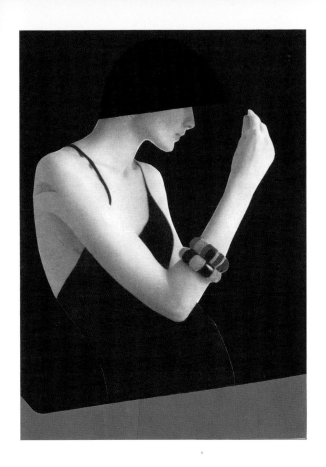

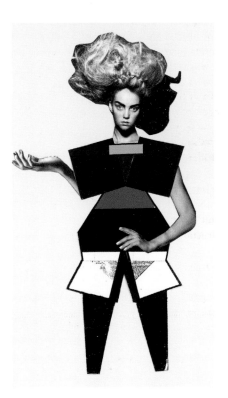

Above, above right and right:
Collages created by Gaia.

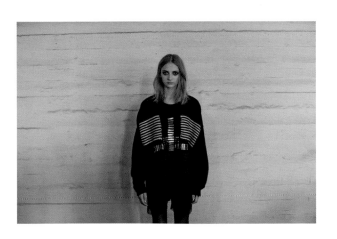

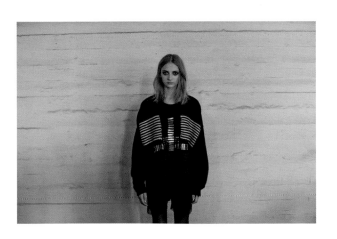

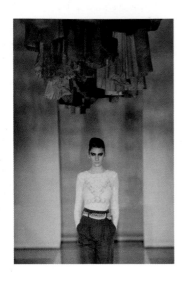

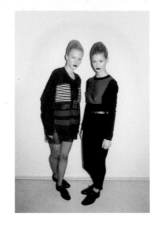

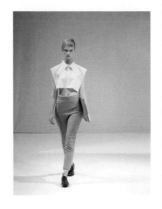

'I like to dabble in colours and graphics from Dadaism and Surrealism'

shops, flea markets and the internet, where I use the imagery quite intuitively. Storytelling is important for my own approach. But I must admit that, though I care a lot about the old virtues and traditions, I don't really consider myself a nostalgic person; rather I enjoy and utilize the details and moods from the photos like a tool to form my shapes.

Tell me about your atelier. Do you sketch? How do you work? The GAIA studio is located in Frederiksberg, a leafy neighbourhood in Copenhagen. Fabric swatches, colourful knits and inspirational pieces surround my workplace. I generally have many things lying around and the walls are full of pictures, collages and samples. I do sketches, but I always

change them in the process of making the garments. For me, designing clothes is an organic process in which one expression leads to another, and suddenly there is a small selection of garments that are well linked together, and the collection takes its more conceptual form gradually.

What is your next step? I aim to develop the GAIA identity and universe in a fresh and clear way, to underline the unmistakable look of the brand. In addition to that, outreach and interaction with our buyers, press and stores are crucial for GAIA. We aim to have a pleasant modus operandi, inspired by an organic and respectful production process, working towards a solid foundation to grow GAIA further internationally.

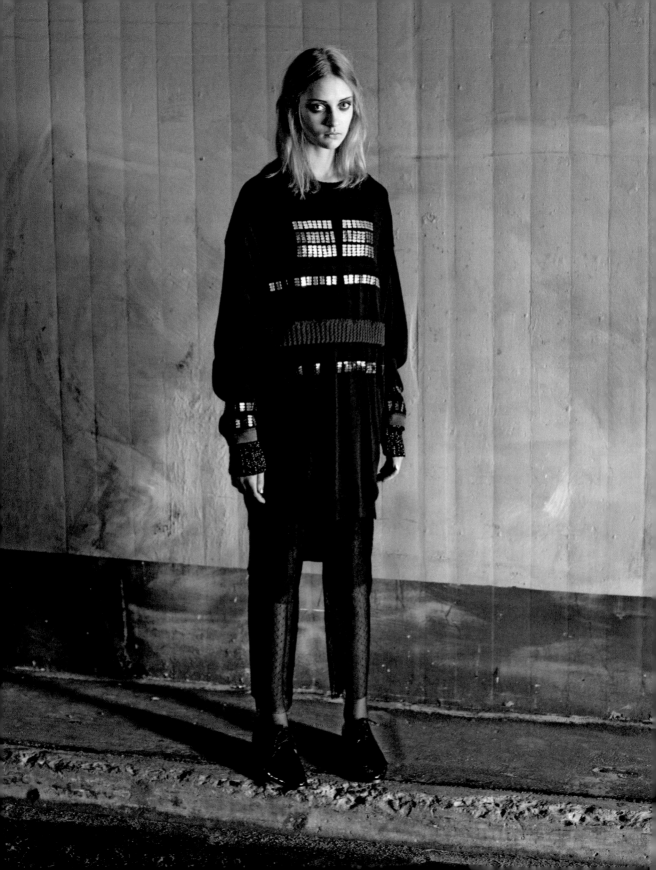

HAANING & HTOON

NORWEGIAN CONCEPTUAL MEETS BRITISH COOL: WHEN FORMER TEACHER MIN HTOON FOUND HIS STAR STUDENT MARIANNE HAANING, THE PERFECT SOLUTION FOR A CONTEMPORARY FASHION DESIGN BRAND WAS BORN. MARIANNE AND MIN'S BACKGROUNDS ALSO TAKE IN EDUCATIONS AT CENTRAL SAINT MARTINS AND ESMOD, AND WORK FOR DOLCE & GABBANA AND ARMANI.

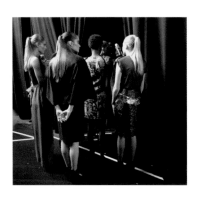
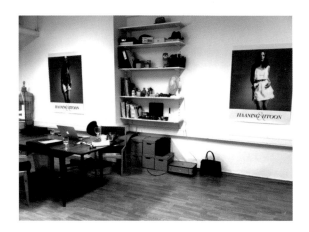

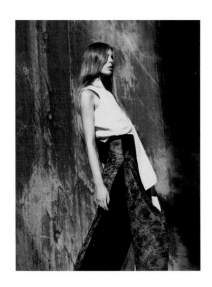
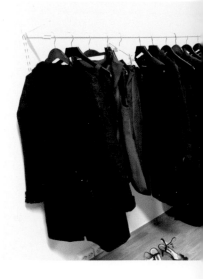

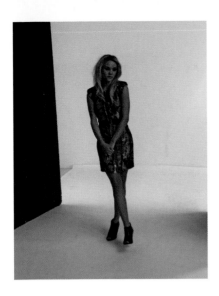

Opposite right and below:
The Haaning & Htoon
studio in Oslo.

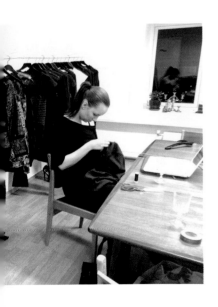

Min, you and Marianne are two designers working together. How did you meet? It's a funny/cute story. I was a teacher at ESMOD in France and Marianne was my star student. We stayed in touch, then when I left my old company the timing was perfect.

What is your background? I graduated from Manchester Metropolitan University with a BA, then an MA from Central Saint Martins. Past international houses I've worked for include Dolce & Gabbana, Donna Karan, Elie Tahari, Armani Exchange and Riccovero. Marianne was a merchandiser/buyer, and she's also worked freelance for various Norwegian and Swedish brands. She's Norwegian-raised but with Danish roots.

Why did you decide to move to Oslo? I love it here. I wanted a change from city life. Going skiing, cycling and hiking … it's hard to do that in Manhattan!

Do you think the British/Scandinavian mix is perfect for understanding the current international market? Definitely. I bring the British Central Saint Martins element and Marianne brings the feminine conceptual. Experience of different markets is invaluable in range-building. I come from a male perspective and Marianne brings the understanding of what a woman wants.

Marianne, you were awarded a Judges' Choice of best collection by Karl Lagerfeld's head of knitwear. Tell me about that experience. I felt it gave me recognition and showed me I was on the right track. This was something I'd wanted to do since I was ten years old.

Min, what would you say your brand is about, and why did you decide to start it? British cool meets Scandinavian conceptual. We were both burning to put our stamp on the world of fashion and felt we had something new to say. With my experience and Marianne's creativity, we felt we had a winning combination. We saw a niche in the market: high quality meeting the right balance of design in a commercially priced product.

You recently won the Norwegian Designer of the Year award. What do you think makes your brand successful? It was amazing winning, when Scandinavian fashion is so big right now. We were judged not only as a creative brand but also as a business. An understanding of where creativity meets the customer's needs was the key, and an ability to execute exactly what we set out to achieve. We also have a more international approach with our brand.

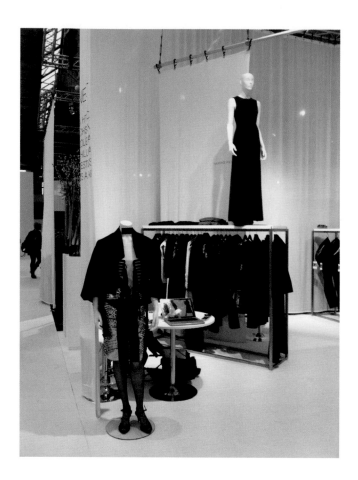

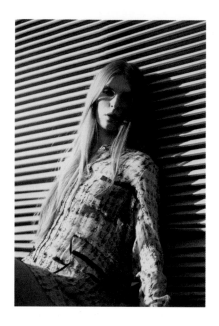

Left: A collection presented during Copenhagen Fashion Week.

Tell me about the inspiration behind your collections.
The theme changes for every season, but our overall inspiration has originated from our many travels and our need for a versatile and functional wardrobe. We've coined it 'the modern traveller'. Norwegian heritage is filled with great explorers and great men and women making their mark. We're inspired by travel and by different cultures meeting and inspiring each other. We also want to bring back pride in dressing up for a journey, like it was in the old days when a trip was a luxury.

What is Scandinavian design to you, and why do you think it is so popular now? Scandinavians are at the mercy of the weather, so nearly everything in their wardrobe has to be practical and functional. They have a phrase: 'There's no such thing as bad weather, only bad clothes.' Scandis have made fashion and functionality meet in an interesting and modern way. Often the colours or the mood have an understated melancholy, as the winters are long and the days are short. The Scandinavians are very inspired by the environment and by their heritage.

What are you working on right now? A launch of a diffusion line for men and women called 'Vandrer' — which in English is 'wanderer'.

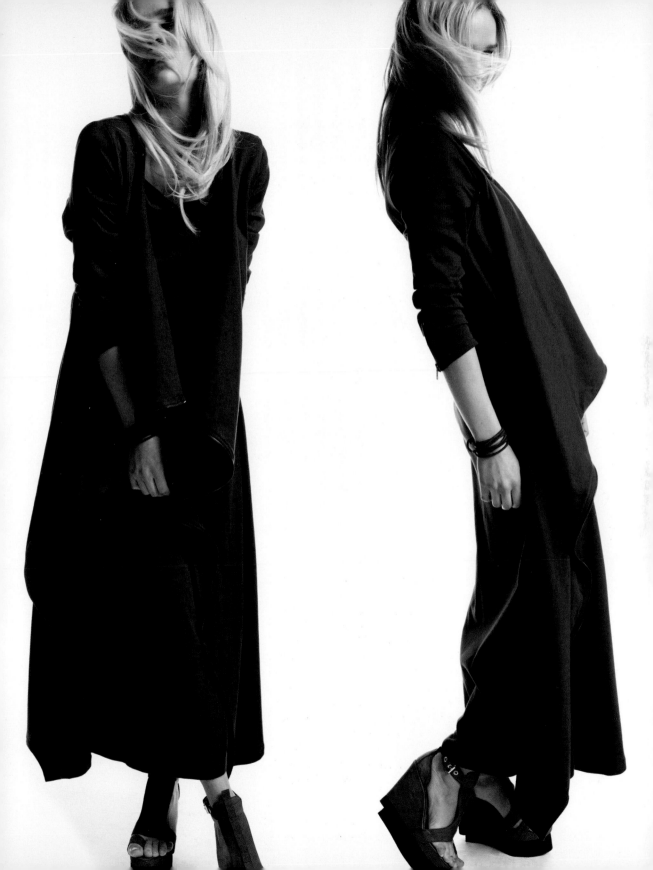

HEIKKI SALONEN

ONE OF FINLAND'S BRIGHTEST FASHION STARS, THIS ROYAL COLLEGE OF ART
GRADUATE WON A COMPETITION JUDGED BY THE DESIGNER ERDEM. THIS RECOGNITION,
TOGETHER WITH SUPPORT FROM FASHION EAST AND NEWGEN, CATAPULTED HIM
ONTO THE INTERNATIONAL FASHION STAGE ... WHICH, IN TURN, OPENED
THE DOOR TO THE HEAD DESIGN POSITION AT DIESEL.

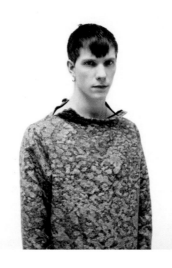

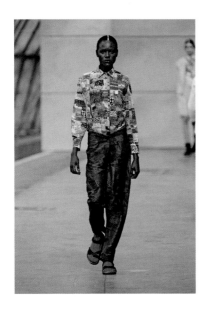

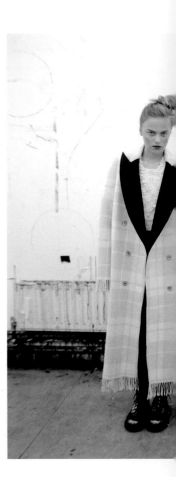

'You can express so many
things through fashion –
social behaviour, politics,
culture...'

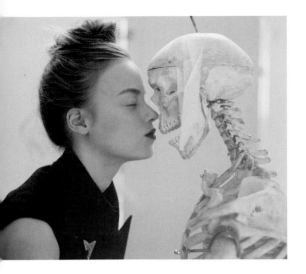

You graduated from the Royal College of Art in London. Can you tell me about your experience of studying there? I really enjoyed my time at the RCA. I was very lucky to have great fellow students, some of whom I've continued to do projects with. Of course the teachers deserve praise, too. The atmosphere was really supportive. I think in our year everybody took the course quite seriously, which I liked a lot.

Did you do any fashion-related studies or work for anyone in your native Finland? I did my BA in Finland. I got into fashion during high school, when I almost accidentally took part in a fashion psychology course at an open university. After that I got a sort of 'good enough' reason to do fashion. You can express so many things through it – social behaviour, politics, cultural environment, etc. It started to make sense.

You have designed for Erdem. Tell me about that process. Erdem was a lecturer in tailoring at the RCA and he was a part of the jury selecting the winners. They gave the prize to me, and I have to say the bigger prize was that a few days later Erdem asked me to join his team for that summer. I did a lot of patterns and fittings and some more constructed, tailored design work. I would have loved to work with him even longer, but I needed to move to Italy.

Your own collection was designed together with the artist Johanna Eliisa Laitanen. How did you find each other and collaborate? Johanna has been my girlfriend for the last eight years. We are partners in work and in love! At the moment we divide most of our time between Italy and Finland, but we still have our studio in London.

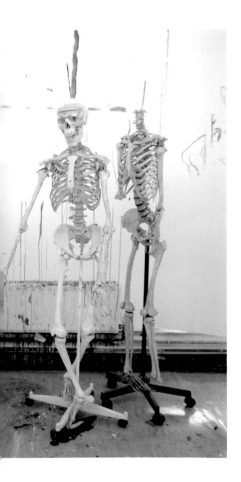

Do you think being a part of the Fashion East show was a good showcase of your work internationally? You, of course, won the Diesel Prize, so that must have helped as well... Both were very important. Everything that happens in life in general is a sum of many things, big and small, and they are all related to each other. For some reason I have met very supportive fashion people, who have helped develop the collection and image.

You are now the head designer at Diesel, but you also have your own brand. How do you manage, time-wise, and where do you design the brands from? I'm lucky to be able to travel a lot, so collection ideas for both lines are developed wherever I am. At the moment, as my job in Diesel is relatively new, I spend more time on the Diesel collection; also the size of it is much bigger.

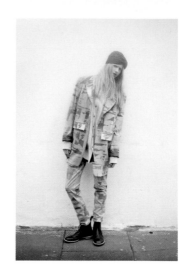

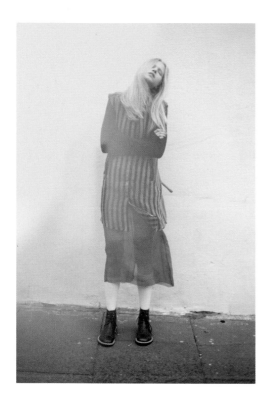

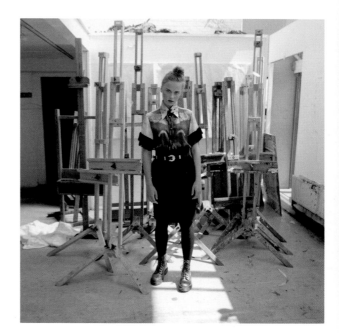

<u>What are you working on at the moment, and for the future?</u> I'm looking forward to a few collaborations that are in the pipeline. I'm actually aiming to make less, while concentrating on quality and finding a real reason for a product to exist in the world. Also I'm really into trying to find a way to develop a collection that's less dependent on a weird fashion cycle. I hope that fashion will soon get its wittiness back and that people will be able to create something poignant again.

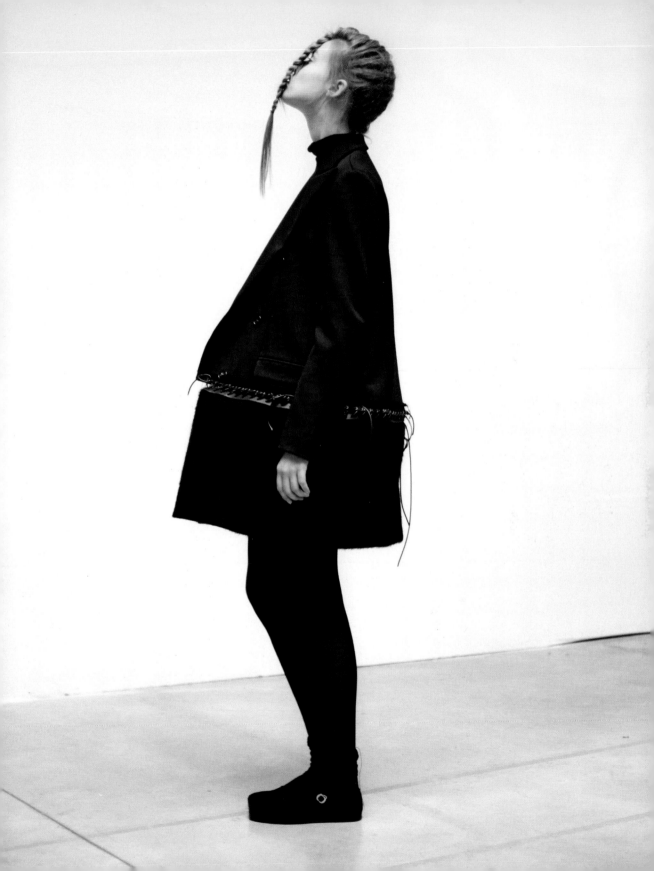

HENRIK VIBSKOV

THIS DANISH DESIGNER SPENDS MORE TIME THINKING ABOUT AND
CREATING HIS PROJECTS THAN SPEAKING ABOUT THEM. HE HIMSELF IS ONE OF THE
MOST TALKED-ABOUT SCANDINAVIAN DESIGNERS AND HAS MANAGED TO ATTRACT
THE LIKES OF FRENCH VOGUE'S EDITOR-IN-CHIEF EMMANUELLE ALT. HE MIXES GIANT
ART-WORLD INSTALLATIONS WITH FASHION PIECES DURING HIS SHOWS AT
COPENHAGEN FASHION WEEK AND MEN'S FASHION WEEK IN PARIS.

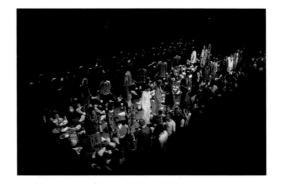

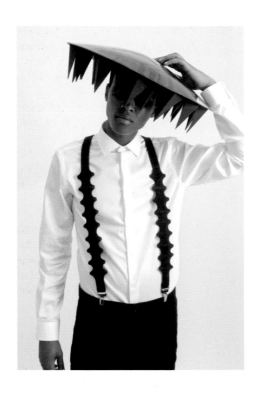

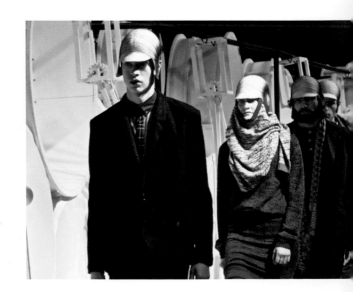

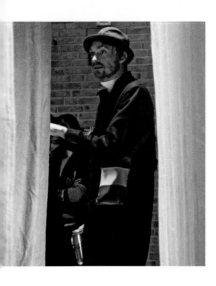

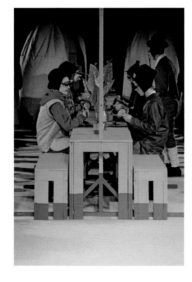

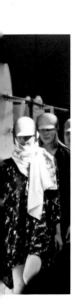

Above: Designer Henrik Vibskov backstage during Copenhagen Fashion Week.

Did you start out by yourself, with no partners? All by myself.

You also play the drums. How do you think you've made art, fashion and music – a dream combination – work together, plus manage to survive on what you love doing? Playing drums is a vital thing for me. I've always had people or bands to play with. For me art, fashion and music emerge from the same source. They're not elements that I manipulate to work together: they're born together, raise each other and co-exist. As for the survival, it's a work-in-progress!

Do you design the collections yourself, or do you employ designers and focus on your art? I do both. I have some design assistants for the fashion collection.

How do you produce those big installations that are always presented with your shows? Is it down to blood, sweat and tears and a huge team? Yep, exactly.

Are you conscious of sustainability and the environment in your work, as many Scandinavian designers seem to be? We try to be as conscious as we can with the materials we choose, the treatments they've had, etc. But this is nothing we communicate loudly; it's just a part of our DNA.

Do you get anything manufactured in Scandinavia, or does everything come from abroad? Our hats are made by a traditional hat-maker in Copenhagen, our socks come from Portugal and our complicated knitwear from Hong Kong. I'm currently trying to manufacture some of our shirts in Peru. Our shoes are from Argentina and our jersey from Turkey. So really it comes from all over the world.

You must travel a lot, what with shops in different cities and probably friends from school living abroad. How do you have time to go on tour, design, make art and prepare a show that is the most anticipated of Copenhagen Fashion Week? Hmmm, I just try not to think about it too much.

You attract people like Emmanuelle Alt from French _Vogue_ to your show in Copenhagen, and she doesn't attend anything else. Are you aware of your concept being watched throughout the world, and was this a goal of yours? Always a goal, never a condition.

What is in store for the future of Henrik Vibskov? Big things in slow motion.

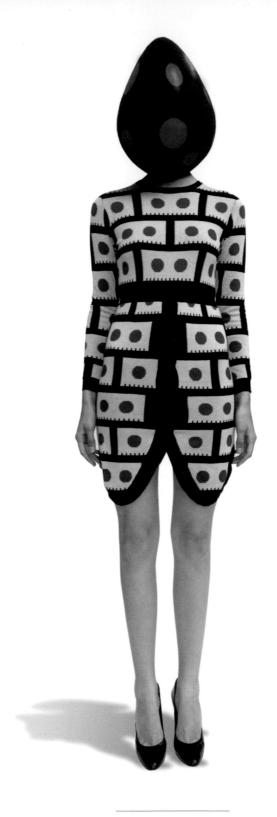

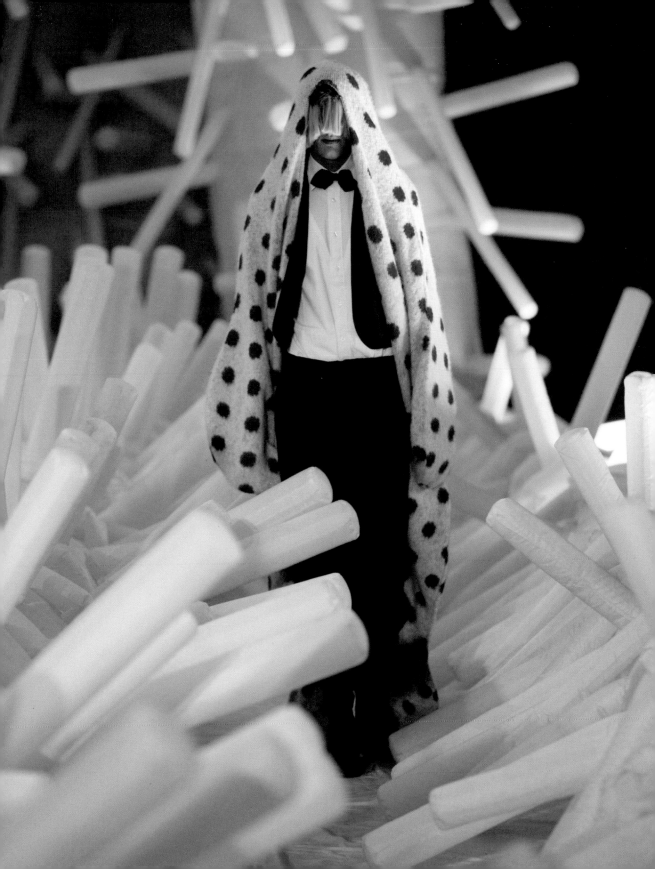

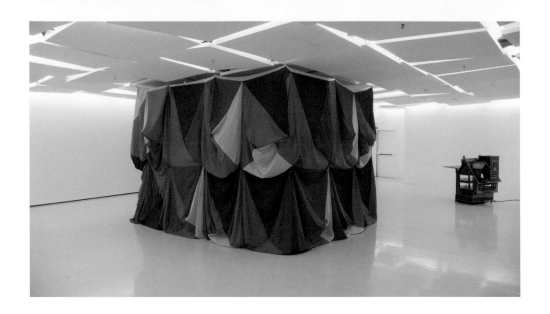

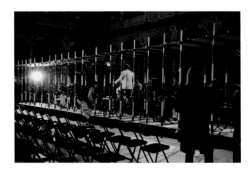

Above: 'Bodybuilding' installation at the Nederlands Architectuurinstituut, Rotterdam.

Below left: Vibskov & Emenius; 'Fringe Project 3 Chairs' for the Mielcke & Hurtigkarl gourmet restaurant, Frederiksberg.

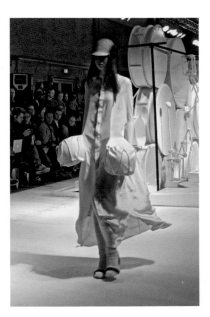

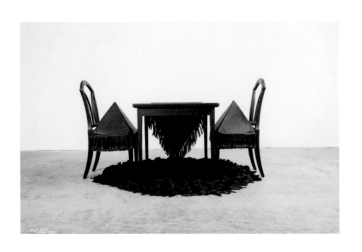

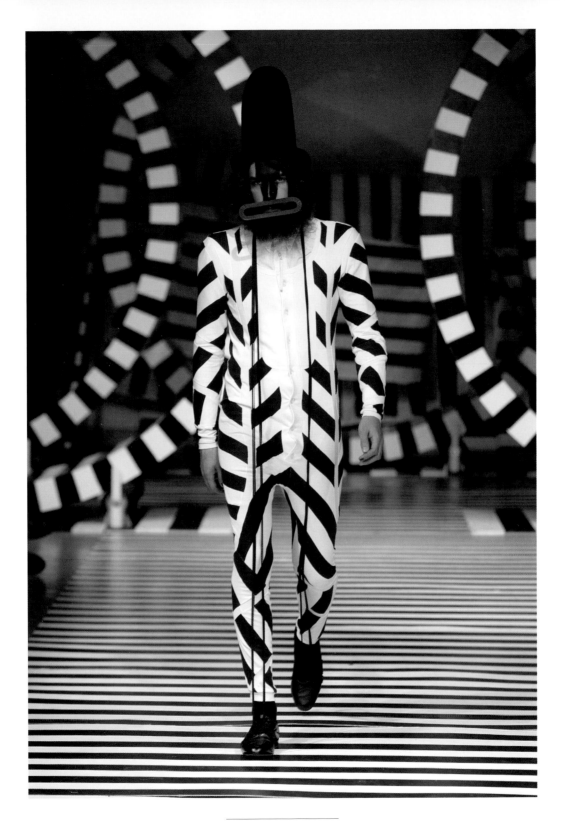

HOPE

THIS AWARD-WINNING SWEDISH LABEL WITH MORE THAN 10 YEARS' EXPERIENCE
ON THE INTERNATIONAL FASHION SCENE IS RUN BY DESIGNERS ANN RINGSTRAND AND
STEFAN SÖDERBERG. THEIR CONCEPT INCLUDES A SOCIAL CONSCIOUSNESS PROJECT, 'STAY
WARM IN YOUR HEART', THAT HAS DONATED PARKAS AND PROFITS TO HOMELESS FAMILIES.
THE COMPANY HAS SEVERAL SHOPS IN SWEDEN AND ONE IN DENMARK.

Ann, how did you and Stefan meet? We both worked at H&M, so we met for the first time there.

You started off with a women's collection in 2001 at the art gallery Björkholmen. What was the idea behind the brand and the word 'Hope'? Our vision was a fashion concept with a special preference for original and classic design. We wanted solid and true engagement for all parts, including the manufacturing process, and we pictured Hope to be an internationally known design label. I had been thinking for quite some time about a brand name, and was looking through an art book and suddenly saw this painting that said 'HOPE' in big letters. I suggested to Stefan that the design label should be 'Let's Hope'. He thought for a while, called me back and said, 'What about just the word "Hope"?'

Did both of you study fashion? Stefan is an autodidact designer. His career started on the retail floor, selling denim. I was brought up in a sewing factory, as my father was running it. My dream was to become a designer and I studied drawing, pattern making and fashion design in Denmark and Sweden's top design schools.

You have to be very good friends to make a company function without quarrels. How does your partnership work? We take on different roles. I am the designer for the women's collection, creative director and CEO, and Stefan's focus lies on designing the men's collection, developing the retail concept and also being creative director. Since we know each other so well, our communication can be totally honest and straightforward. We use each other as the first critical barrier to test new ideas. In the end we always come up with the strongest ideas together.

One of the things that has really impressed me is your social consciousness project, which I think all brands should do. Tell me a bit more about it. As soon as we had the opportunity financially, we wanted to contribute and take social responsibility by using our skills outside of the company. One of the things we do well is warm and durable outerwear, and sharing that with Stockholms Stadsmission felt warm in our hearts.

You have people like Nina Persson from The Cardigans, singer Lykke Li and actor Alexander Skarsgård involved in the project. What is their main responsibility? They are all from time to time ambassadors for Hope, which in general means that we approve of each other's values and support the need for a coup. One of our offers to the ambassadors is to be a part of the 'Stay Warm In Your Heart' project and to support our engagement to help with homes for homeless young families and also to prevent homelessness.

You call your garments 'utility wear' and it seems more important for you to design comfortable clothes than to design couture wear. Why did you decide that this should be the focus of the company? We love the look of utility wear worn in a fashionable way, both by men and women. I'm thinking parkas, car coats, blazers, jackets, tailored men's trousers… This style is quite common for men, but for women we picture the look with open feminine sandals and thin blouses. Our passion lies with designs that are inspired by uniforms and tailoring in a very relaxed way. We focus on details and fine material development rather than on grand colourful runway pieces. We love designing for everyday life. Luckily at the time we started, this look was also missing on the market, so we saw a potential business opportunity.

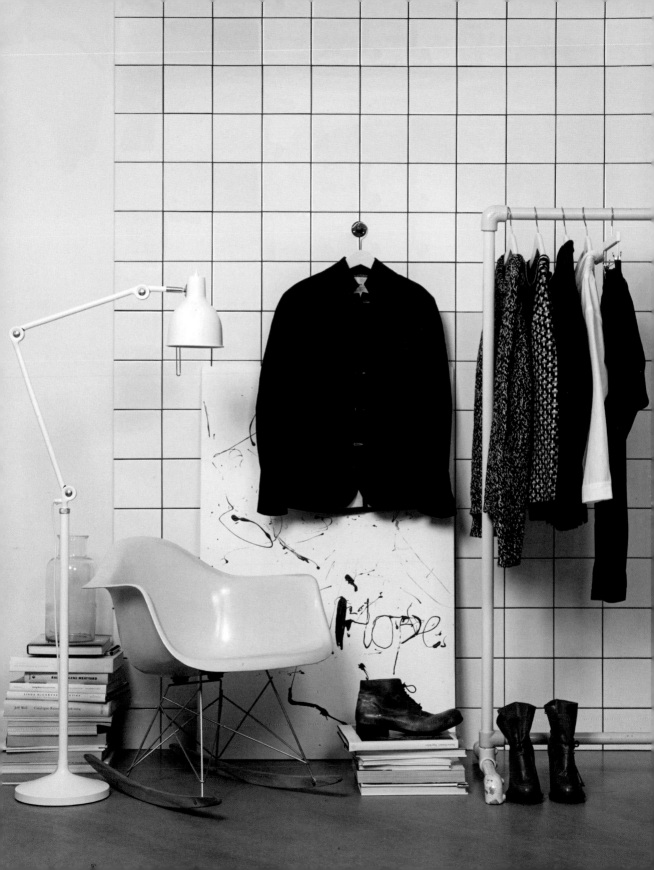

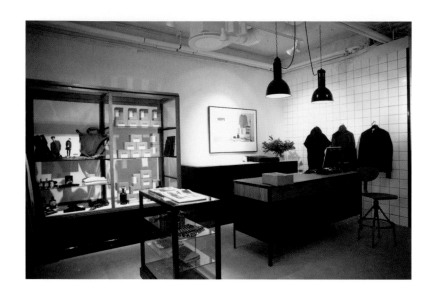

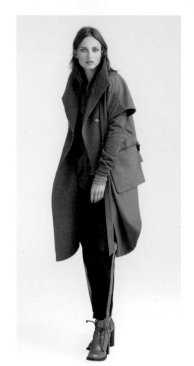

Above: Hope shop
in Stockholm.

Below right: A close-up
of print fabric.

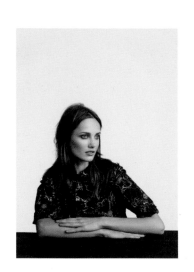

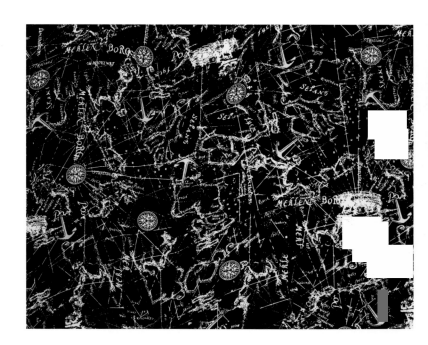

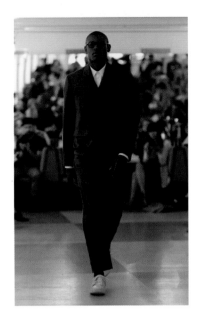

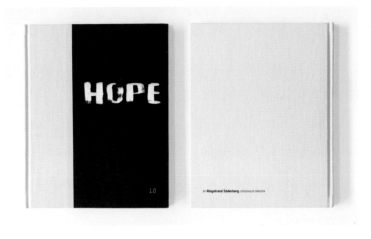

I remember being at a presentation you held in your shop in Copenhagen; I think it was a collaboration with the magazine _Cover_. How have things changed since then? The big challenge is to spread the vision, feeling and culture of Hope on to all co-workers. Another change is in brand awareness. I find it hard to believe but there are a lot of people out there, all over the world, who have a relationship with Hope today, as a result of many years of hard work.

Which international stores carry Hope? A selection of stores includes Bungalow in Stuttgart, Set & Sekt in Basel, Barneys and Project No. 8 in New York, Steven Alan in New York, San Francisco and Los Angeles, Isetan Mitsukoshi and Desperado in Tokyo, La Garçonne online in the States, Margriet Nannings and SPRMRKT in Amsterdam, and You Are Here in Eindhoven, to name but a few.

Tell me about your design process. Where do you find inspiration, and where are your garments manufactured? There's a constant flow of ideas and inspiration in our minds and in our creative studio. It's not only about the collection itself; it's also about the concept, the communication and the Hope shops. We collect ideas four times a year to be the basis for a new collection. Stefan is more into the materials and colours, and I'm more into the context and the design. We discuss ideas, do workshops and travel when it's time for the hardcore collection structure, delivery windows and updated fit and function in proto-development. We make our garments mainly in Europe and the Far East at smaller factories with high-quality skills and a good code of conduct.

Do you think you convey that you are inspired by the modern Scandinavian woman in your designs? I think we create and supply an opportunity for the modern Scandinavian woman to dress in an updated way for an everyday purpose and with a creative expression. Our design comes from this need within ourselves more than from speculation as to what someone else might want.

HOUSE OF DAGMAR

THREE SWEDISH SISTERS DESIGN UNDER A NAME INSPIRED BY THEIR LATE GRANDMOTHER, DAGMAR. THEY HAVE WON SOME OF SCANDINAVIA'S MOST RESPECTED AWARDS AND CAUGHT THE EYE OF ACCLAIMED FASHION JOURNALIST HILARY ALEXANDER. THE SISTERS – KRISTINA TJÄDER, KARIN SÖDERLIND AND SOFIA WALLENSTAM – PUT THEIR HEART AND SOUL, AND GREAT ATTENTION TO DETAIL, INTO THEIR DESIGNS.

Tell me about your beginning in 2005. We started with a ten-piece collection consisting only of knits. We worked from Kristina's basement for the first two years. Her mother-in-law came over every time we got deliveries to help us sort everything out for our customers. The first year we delivered everything to the stores ourselves. For each season the collection grew a little bit. We all had two jobs at the same time for the first year.

You call your design philosophy 'arty chic'. What does this mean to you? It means that our design is based on classic styles and silhouettes, but is never conventional. You can expect typical Dagmar features in each and every garment. 'Sophisticated' is to us always endeavouring to work with luxurious fabrics and to have production of the best quality.

I saw your show in Stockholm. Hilary Alexander and I were almost fighting to have a closer look at that knitwear. So beautiful! Where does it come from? Our knitwear is produced in Europe and we use only the nicest Italian yarns. We started with knitwear and it is close to our hearts in many ways – from the very heavy yarns with a funky appearance to the very fine yarns in the 'prêt-à-couture' collection, which has extremely exclusive production. We design the lace ourselves and then leave it with a factory, and the technicians work for a long time installing all the design details into the machines, then they knit it in one piece, which is fantastic workmanship and based on tradition and lots of knowledge. We saw rugs and other interiors items as inspiration at the beginning, but also furs and woven 'red carpet' kinds of dresses.

You are three sisters running the company. How do you split up the different jobs that have to be done?

Do you all have a design background? Sofia is the youngest; she was only 21 when we started. She's been in charge of sales since the beginning and is now in charge of starting up new markets. Kristina was educated at ESMOD in Paris and is our head of design. Karin was a buyer at H&M for many years and is now in charge of marketing.

Kristina, you worked for Christian Lacroix in Paris and you've also worked for H&M. Those two are like opposites. Do you think having them in your background gives you a certain mix of couture and mainstream? It's definitely given me a good base, having worked with both smaller brands and a large H&M. But we have always had a desire for high quality, and therefore when starting Dagmar we chose to make our dream clothes.

Who inspires your design? Do you have a muse? Our first muse was our grandmother, Dagmar: we always have her in mind. But lots of people inspire us – more in their personalities or their way of living than in their form of clothing. We really try to find the modern woman's way of dressing and her needs, and we try to be very contemporary in our minds.

You have won several awards, from the 2005 'Rookie of the Year' from the Swedish Fashion Council to the 2011 Guldknappen, which is Scandinavia's most prestigious design award. What do you think makes your design so accessible and successful? I think it's that we don't follow anyone or anything. We feel quite confident about what we want and what we like. If we see a trend coming, we never jump on it. We find it very important to stick to what Dagmar is about, and not do what everyone else is doing. Swedish *Elle* said we are 'the contrary sisters'. Kind of like that...

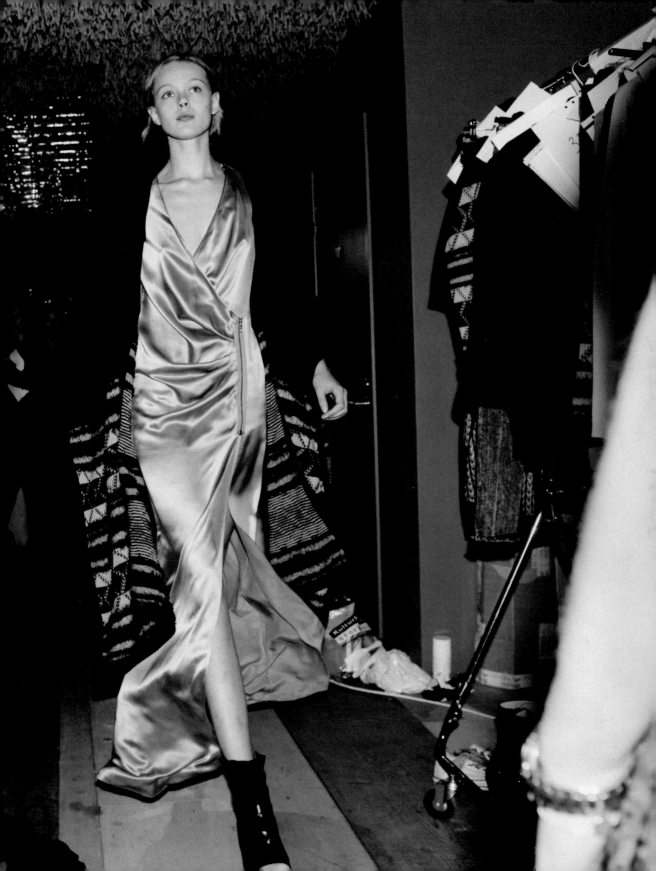

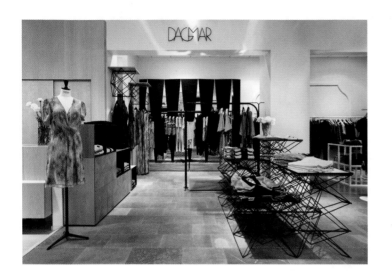

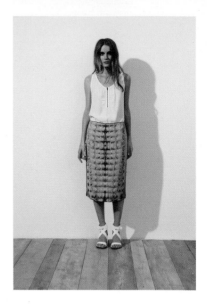

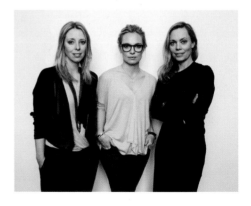

Above: House of Dagmar shop in Stockholm.

Right: Designer sisters Kristina Tjäder, Karin Söderlind and Sofia Wallenstam.

'Our design is based on classic styles and silhouettes, but is never conventional'

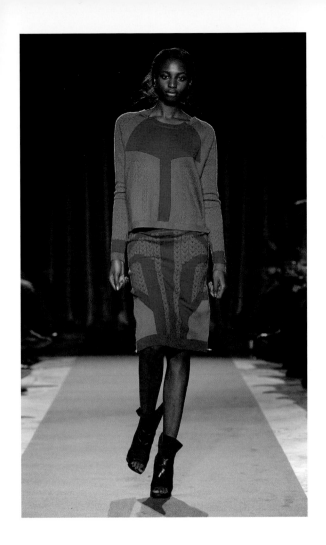

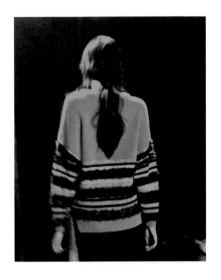

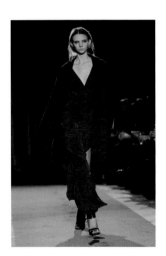

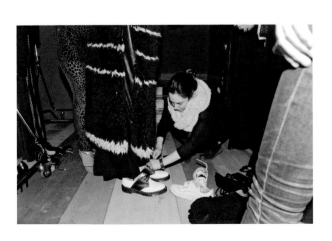

IDA SJÖSTEDT

THIS SWEDISH DESIGNER GRADUATED FROM THE UNIVERSITY OF WESTMINSTER AND INTERNED AT JOHN RICHMOND AND DAI REES BEFORE STARTING HER OWN LABEL, SHOWCASED IN PARIS AND COPENHAGEN. SHE MEETS WITH HER COUTURE CLIENTS IN PERSON, WHICH NO DOUBT EXPLAINS WHY HER HANDMADE COLLECTIONS HAVE BECOME SO POPULAR IN SWEDEN AND THE REST OF THE WORLD.

You graduated in fashion design from the University of Westminster. What was it like studying there, and why didn't you study at a Scandinavian school? I first studied fashion in high school in Sweden, but there wasn't any real fashion scene here back then. When visiting London, I fell in love with the city and decided I wanted to continue my studies there. I started with a foundation at London College of Fashion and then I visited all the top five colleges of the time – Central Saint Martins, Westminster, Kingston, Middlesex and Ravensbourne – and Westminster seemed to be the perfect match for me. I liked the facilities, and the course director Nigel [Luck] had great charisma, and I felt it would be the best place for me to study. That also made me confident at my interview, as I already knew I had made the right choice.

Did you do any internships along the way? I interned at John Richmond and Dai Rees and, after graduating, I worked part-time for six months in the design studios of Dai Rees, Marcus Constable and high-end T-shirt label On the Subject Of.

What have you been working on since your graduation? At On the Subject Of I was design assistant and pattern cutter, and I also checked some production in London. With Dai Rees I mainly sewed in their studio for the show at London Fashion Week. At Marcus Constable I was a part-time design assistant, mainly running the work in the studio, sourcing fabrics, etc. It wasn't good pay but I learned a lot in all three places about how to run a small design-based studio, like the one I now run myself.

Where do you exhibit your collection during Paris Fashion Week? How does it give you a better platform for sales than clients visiting Scandinavia? I used to meet clients in Paris at hotels, but the last few seasons I have actually been doing 'Gallery' in Copenhagen instead of Paris.

What kind of stores carry your designs? Mainly multiple-brand stores who carry other Scandinavian and/or international designer labels, but also some department stores, and more and more webstores, from big ones like nelly.com to smaller boutiques like 30 Cancan.

You also create a couture line. What kind of clients do you have for this? Are they mostly Swedish? It's mostly brides-to-be, ordering wedding dresses. We mainly have Swedish customers, but I've also made dresses for clients in Denmark, Norway, Switzerland, the USA and Australia.

Tell me about the approach of creating these dresses. I've always had a few hand-worked showpieces in my collections, but the stores we sell to couldn't really buy them. Customers started requesting them, so we started doing some private orders, and since then it's grown. I have a small office/showroom in Stockholm, where I meet all my clients personally and show them our range of approximately ten dresses – from various seasons, as we want these to be more timeless than the ready-to-wear collection. It's been really nice for me to be able to sell these pieces, which are so much more worked than the ready-to-wear.

Do you create your couture gowns completely in the studio from scratch with no help, or do you have a team? We make them from scratch. For the embroidered crystals we order pieces that are embroidered out in India but we then cut and attach everything by hand onto each dress in the studio. When we make our own prints, we make the design in

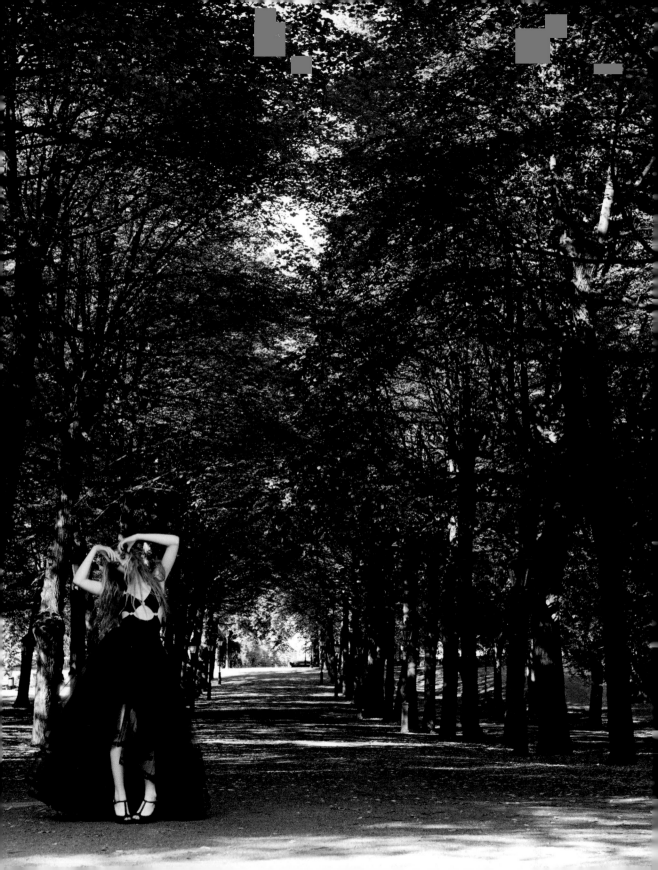

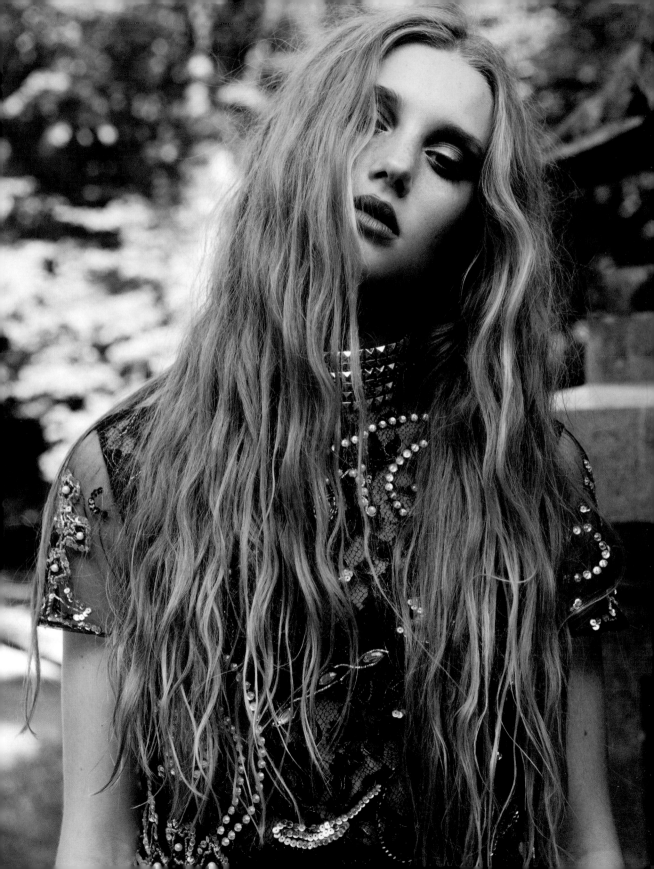

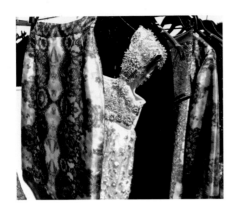

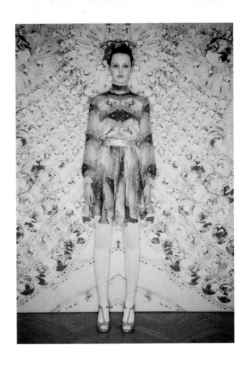

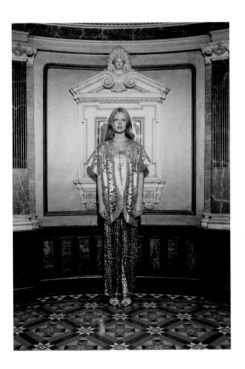

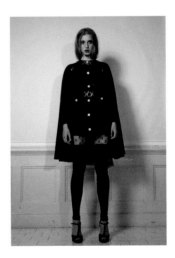

the studio, but then of course we have the print produced by a printer. Each dress is, however, cut and sewn from scratch by me and my team in the studio.

<u>What do you think about Scandinavian design today?</u>
<u>Does it influence your design?</u> I like Scandinavian design and I'm proud of being a Scandinavian designer. I wouldn't say I'm influenced by other Scandinavian designers, though, as I've always felt much more connected to London designers in terms of aesthetics, concepts and how we work in the studio … and I've also always been more inspired by the couture houses in Paris, in terms of craftsmanship.

IVAN GRUNDAHL

HE IS ONE OF THE MOST RECOGNIZABLE AND LONG-LIVED OF DESIGNERS.
HIS AVANT-GARDE SHOPS WERE THE GO-TO FASHION BOUTIQUES FOR THE POST-PUNK CROWD
IN COPENHAGEN IN THE LATE 1980S. HE SEEMS TO WORK IN THE SAME MANNER AS
JUNYA WATANABE AND OTHERS OF THE JAPANESE SET, DESPITE HIS SCANDINAVIAN
ROOTS AND A SELF-PROCLAIMED 'NORMAL' BACKGROUND.

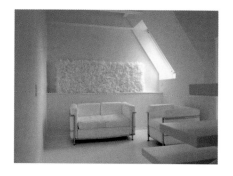

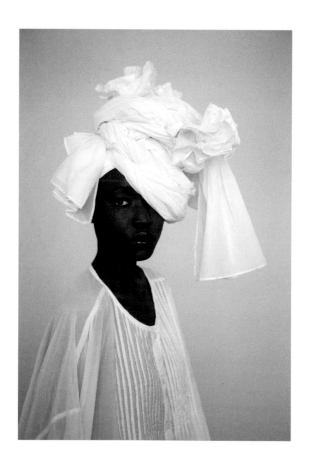

Above: The Ivan Grundahl
atelier.

Below: Shop in Copenhagen.

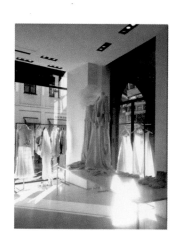

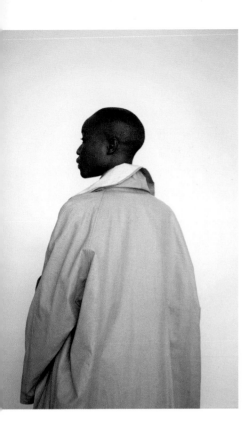

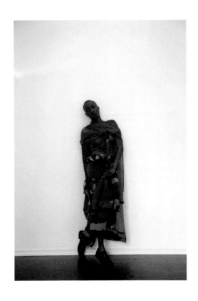

Tell me about your upbringing. Did you grow up in a creative environment? No, I grew up in a very normal family in Denmark!

Where does your design style come from? Is there any particular architecture or movement that has inspired you? I'm normally inspired by architects such as Mies van der Rohe, or Japanese designers such as Yohji Yamamoto, Junya Watanabe, Comme des Garçons…

When did you start out in fashion and how did it happen? Did you work for a designer or did you go through the design school system? I worked at the fashion shop Birger Christensen at the same time as attending the Royal Danish Design School.

Your stores are pretty spectacular. They light up a street, especially in Scandinavia, where it is often dark. When did you come up with the concept? I always just look around everywhere I am, but mostly in big cities such as New York.

In fact you opened a shop in New York as well. Have you ever lived there? The lifestyle in New York is always interesting to me. I go there on and off all the time.

Do you design the whole collection yourself, or do you have a team around you? Sometimes I do, sometimes I don't; depends on what it is.

Where are the garments produced? Anything in Denmark? Not in Denmark; our production units are in Portugal, Italy, India and Bulgaria.

You have been doing this for many years but have now decided to launch a menswear line. How come? Just to have a little bit of fun and to do something completely new – for me, at least.

You are quite different from the other Scandinavian designers and seem to keep yourself a bit on the outside, although you still present your collection during Copenhagen Fashion Week. Have you ever showcased in Paris instead? We show our collections in Denmark, Norway and the USA – no more now.

Apart from the new menswear line, do you have anything else coming up? You never know with me!

IVANA HELSINKI

ARTIST, FILM MAKER AND FASHION DESIGNER ARE JUST SOME OF THE TITLES APPLICABLE TO THE FINNISH DESIGNER PAOLA SUHONEN. SHE LIVES AND WORKS IN LOS ANGELES, WHERE SHE STUDIES FILM AT THE AMERICAN FILM INSTITUTE. SHE HAS AN OFFICE IN HELSINKI AND SHOWS DURING NEW YORK FASHION WEEK; IN 2007, IVANA HELSINKI WAS ALSO THE FIRST FINNISH COMPANY EVER TO PARTICIPATE IN PARIS FASHION WEEK. EVEN THOUGH HER COMPANY IS HIGHLY SUCCESSFUL AND EXPANDING RAPIDLY, PAOLA KEEPS HER FEET ON THE GROUND BY CAPTURING MOMENTS ON HER ANALOGUE CAMERA.

When one first opens your website, one gets sucked into a universe of travel, dreams and imagination. You really combine it all beautifully. Where does this world come from? It's the world in my own head. It's a mixture of lived life, dreams, hopes and fairy tales. I know this world exists – it's all about angels, champagne, love stories, dark forests, clear lakes, drummer girls – and all of my designs are just souvenirs from this world. The world itself is the soul for all of this.

You combine Slavic blood with Scandinavian calm. Tell me about your upbringing. I grew up in the most loving family, with my sister who's one year older, in Helsinki. My mom's family comes from Russia (her grandmother was a famous Russian fortune-teller, who worked for the Tsar). I guess my love of Slavic aesthetics comes from there. My dad comes from a really typical Scandinavian countryside family, for whom nature was part of the simple rural lifestyle. I've always loved both of those cultures but I've also always mixed urban culture and a hint of an Americana vintage flavour into my imaginary world. I love camping, road trips, dark winters, melancholic autumns and huge love stories. I was supposed to be a snowboarder when I was a teenager, and I travelled around the world and lived kind of a hippie life doing that. I've always hated fashion but loved the poetic, bohemian life.

Did you study to become a fashion designer, or did you start out as an artist? I started as an artist, then did my MA in fashion, and now I'm back to my roots, studying cinema, telling stories.

You made a beautiful film, with an almost Jim Jarmusch 'Night on Earth' tenderness. How do you have time to go on road trips, make films, take photographs and manage a whole collection? Thanks, that's a great compliment! Yes, 7 *Heaven LoveWays* is my film, a collaboration with my all-time favourite, Chip Taylor – he's so cool! And, yes, I love Jim Jarmusch. I guess it's all about my passion, the way of life. I've never considered my work as 'work'; it's more like just living and being on an adventure. Of course it's sometimes a lot of work, but if you have a passion, a mission, it's something you just can't stop doing.

Why did you decide to translate your artwork into pieces of clothing? I love the idea of pop culture; art blending with something more commercial and a part of everyday life. I've always loved cute dresses, and there are never enough of them! If a dress is like a piece of art, it's above fashion or trends. It's something you love and want to tell a story of who you are. It's also the most ecological way of designing – doing something that never loses its value and is never 'last season'. That's a thing about fashion and fashionistas that makes me sick.

Do you work from Finland in an office space with a big team, or at home? How do you prefer to prepare a collection? I live in Los Angeles now, in Silverlake. I have my old house with a garden and fruit trees, my dog, my coffee machine, a lot of natural light, my candles, and my huge desk and Macs. This is my studio, my world for designing. The rest of the Ivana Helsinki team is in Helsinki and New York. Here I'm alone, and I do miss home, but LA is the Americana road-trip

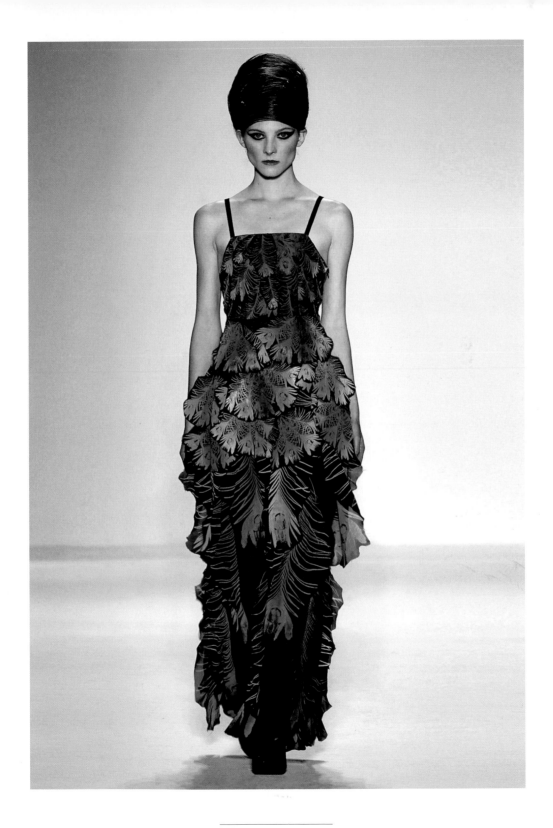

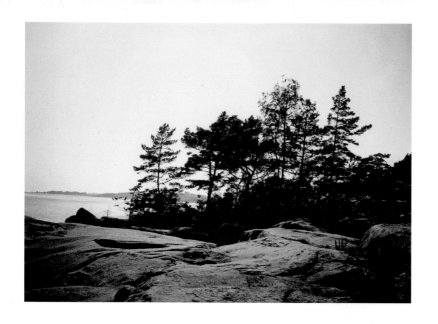

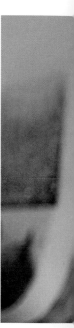

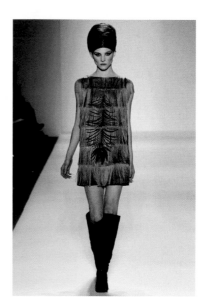

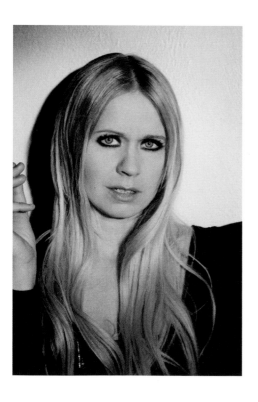

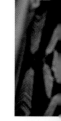

Left: Designer Ivana Helsinki.

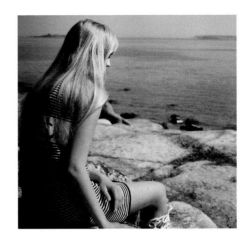

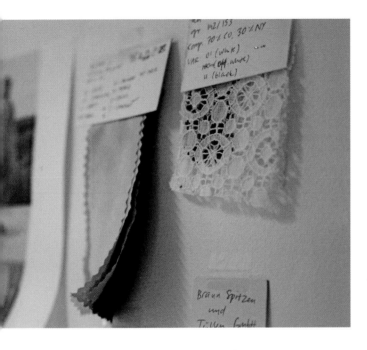

'It's the world in my own head.
It's a mixture of lived life, dreams,
hopes and fairy tales'

ON INSPIRATION

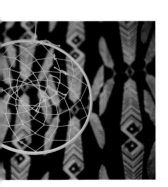

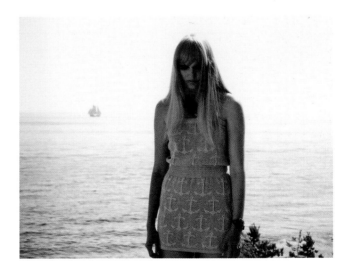

'If a dress is like a piece of art, it's above fashion or trends. It's something you love and want to tell a story of who you are'

ON DESIGN

town, the place where Route 66 ends or starts, however you want to put it, and, yes, I'm here because of the film school where I'm finishing my Masters right now.

You seem to have collaborated with a lot of different brands, including HP Sauce, Topshop, Coca-Cola, a smoke alarm, even a furniture company. How did these collaborations come about? I feel lucky, as all of those were request design collaborations, meaning that someone saw my world and felt it was something they wanted to explore as well with their products, designs or brands. I got a free hand to play with them!

Tell me about the manufacturing process. Where do the garments come from? We have our own atelier in downtown Helsinki, with a lot of old sewing machines from my dad's old jeans factory, so we have our own production. Bigger series come from Lithuania. All the fabrics are designed by me and they are printed in Italy and Portugal. Knits are manufactured by a small family company in southern Finland. We want to keep the production ecological and ethical; really feel it and be part of the handcraft.

Yours is the only Scandinavian womenswear brand to be accepted into the official Paris Fashion Week '"IN" Show' calendar. That must take some nerve! How do you think the Scandinavian market differs from the scene in Paris? It's a different world. We are like northern hippies, as Paris is like *the* fashion capital and Scandinavians are more down-to-earth when it comes to fashion or design – practical but bohemian and experimental.

Where are your collections available from? We have our own three stores – two in Helsinki and one in New York – then we also sell throughout the world, from small boutiques to department stores. I guess we are in fifteen countries now…

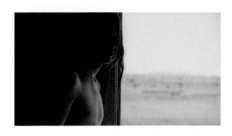

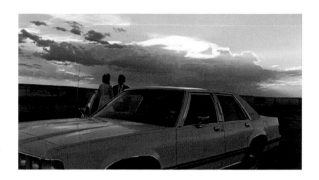

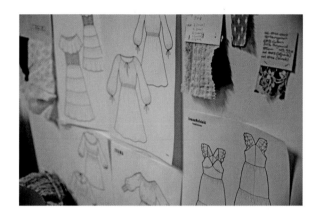

<u>Above left and right:</u>
Stills from '7 Heaven Love Ways', a film by Ivana Helsinki.

<u>Below:</u> The atelier workshop in Helsinki.

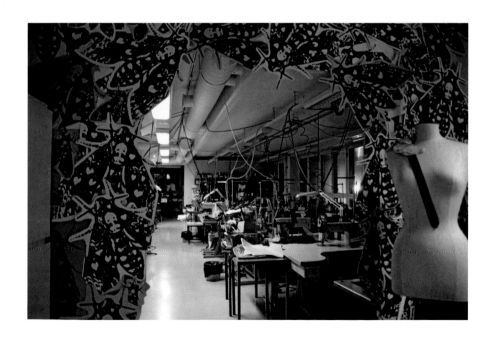

J.LINDEBERG

THIS GIANT SWEDISH BRAND WITH A SUCCESSFUL GOLF LINE BROKE THE RULES IN 2002 BY CHOOSING TO PRESENT A COLLECTION DURING NEW YORK FASHION WEEK. IT HAS LAUNCHED SHOPS ACROSS THE WORLD AND ENJOYED MANY SUCCESSFUL CREATIVE COLLABORATIONS. AS A MODERN INTERNATIONAL BRAND, IT PROGRESSIVELY BRIDGES FASHION WITH FUNCTION.

Malin [Odelfelt], as PR and Marketing Manager, can you tell me about the beginning of J.Lindeberg? The company was founded in 1996 in Stockholm. The vision was to build an international brand for the modern, aware consumer. The first collection was presented in 1997 and featured men's fashion and golfwear. J.Lindeberg launched a small revolution in the relatively conservative golf environment through progressive designs and sponsorships. With quick growth, the company established itself in Scandinavia, North America, Europe and Asia.

How did you break out of Scandinavia? With an outspoken vision to reach international markets, the company opened a flagship store in New York in 2001 and presented its collection at Bryant Park during New York Fashion Week in 2002. New York was followed by Milan, where J.Lindeberg first showed – AW03 – at Milano Moda Uomo Fashion Week.

How would you describe yourselves as a Scandinavian brand and identity? J.Lindeberg is positioned as the fashion house from Scandinavia that bridges fashion and function, offering outstanding products with a high sense of fashion awareness and quality. It has a sleek, precise, sporty silhouette – always with a sense of effortless elegance, which is very Scandinavian. It also has a progressive take on tailoring, fusing the worlds of fashion, golf and skiing, for an active, modern man or woman.

You have used Juliette Lewis and Alison Mosshart as models. Why did you choose them? Campaigns, sponsorships and artistic collaborations have always been a strong focus for J.Lindeberg. Our biannual book project, *The Documentary and the Dream*, started in 2009. Twice a year we produce this

large-format book with the ambition of capturing the inner spirit of the collections. Each season we collaborate with talented photographers, writers, illustrators and artists, such as Olivier Zahm, Andreas Sjödin, Robbie Spencer, Ben Toms, Skye Parrott and Peter Lindbergh, to name but a few. The book is printed in a limited edition of six hundred and is available to read in the J.Lindeberg stores and on the website.

Who is the head designer at J.Lindeberg today? Jessy Heuvelink, who has been with the company for seven years. He was previously at Christian Lacroix and Adidas. He stepped into the position of head designer in 2011.

Do you consider it important/essential for the brand to branch out into different parts of the world? It's always been important for the brand to present the collections in its own retail environment. Flagship stores are today to be found in cities like Stockholm, Copenhagen, New York, Los Angeles, Miami, Hong Kong, Singapore, Seoul, Tokyo and Osaka. J.Lindeberg apparel is also carried by leading independent boutiques, upscale department stores and some of the world's most exclusive golf and ski shops.

Tell me about your work base and the future. The company's headquarters are in Stockholm, with the office situated just by the water in the old Customs House, a beautiful Art Nouveau building designed by Swedish architect Ferdinand Boberg in 1906. With new owners from 2011, the company is looking at an exciting future, with continuous growth in new markets, ready to take on the world!

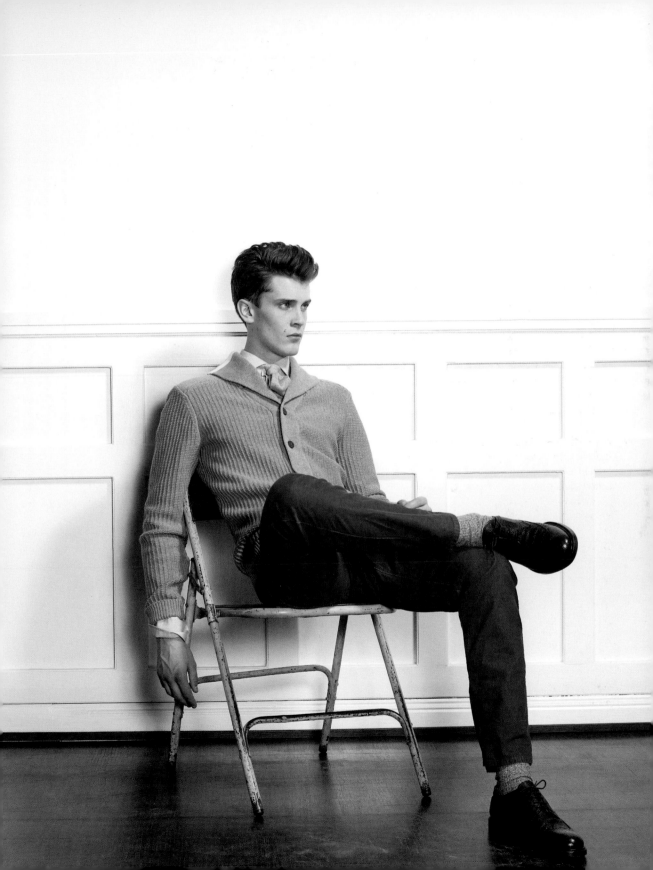

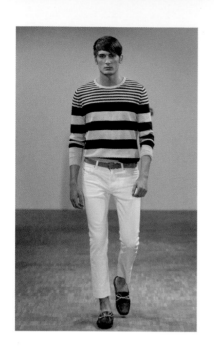

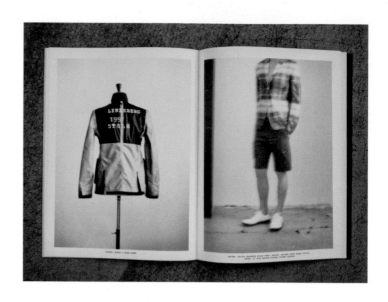

'A sleek, precise, sporty silhouette –
always with a sense of effortless
elegance, which is very Scandinavian'

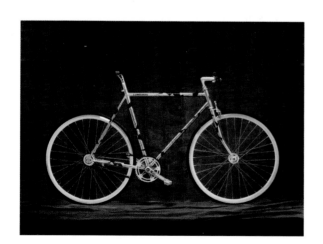

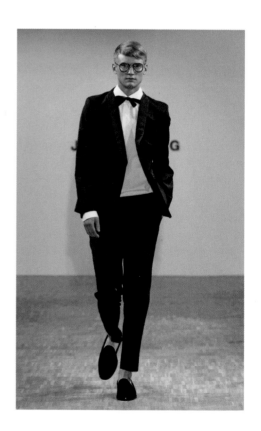

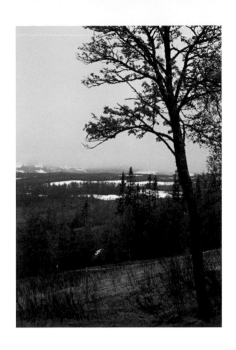

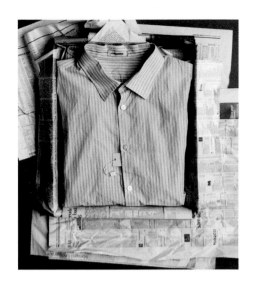

'A progressive take on tailoring,
fusing the worlds of fashion,
golf and skiing, for an active,
modern man or woman'

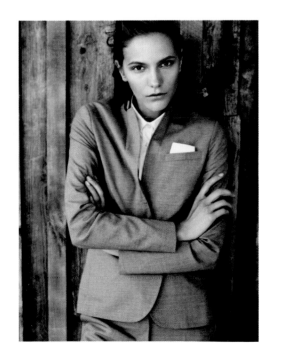

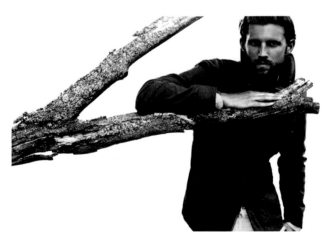

JEAN PHILLIP

HE MIGHT HAVE GROWN UP IN THE DARK COUNTRYSIDE OF DENMARK,
BUT DURING PARIS FASHION WEEK HIS COLLECTIONS ARE SNAPPED UP BY STORES
IN JAPAN AND AMERICA. HIS MENSWEAR IS ALSO SHOWCASED AT COPENHAGEN
FASHION WEEK. HE IS PROOF THAT THE SELF-TAUGHT HAVE SOME ADVANTAGES
OVER THE MORE SCHOOLED SET, IN THAT THEIR CREATIVE PROCESSES
ARE NOT LIMITED WHEN MANUFACTURING.

Tell me about your upbringing in Denmark. I grew up in the countryside, on the dark side of Jutland. I always had a passion for different things from the boys I grew up around, so I spent a lot of time by myself, drawing and dreaming. I've always been a loner, and still am. I love my friends and my husband, but I also need space for thinking and creating.

Like Silas Adler [see p. 210], you haven't been schooled into a stereotype. Do you think this has been one of your strengths? No doubt it's been a strength, as it makes me have no limits when it comes to creating. Others stop along the way because they've learned the 'right' ways of doing things at school, whereas if I set my mind to something I push until it gets to where I want it to be, no matter how it's created.

When and why did you decide you were going to set up on your own? I tried to get into design school in Denmark three times. After the third attempt I got so tired of a school dictating whether or not I was capable of being a designer that I ended up taking fate into my own hands to prove them wrong.

How did you learn everything? Handling materials, patterns, business… I was born handy. It's never been an issue, as it was something that came logically to me.

Do you plan on expanding your company so that one day you're based somewhere other than Denmark? In time it would be lovely to be more settled in Paris, but I'm in no hurry.

What has been one of your career highlights so far, and how long have you had your own label now? The biggest highlight for me is to be able to design so selfishly and still be able to make a living from it! The label has existed since 2007.

Is every piece handmade and checked by you, then sent off to the factory? Tell me about your daily process. Every piece goes through me, but with the collections amounting to eighty styles a season so far it would be hard without assistance. I draw the collection, source materials and create patterns on my own, then either I or my assistants sew the samples. During this process 30% of the collection gets made in factories – that is, if we want to create a style that has a special wash or dye that we aren't able to create ourselves. Apart from that, there are a lot of calls and emails.

Whereabouts in Paris do you showcase your collection? Do you do your own sales? I showcase at a private showroom in Paris and at fairs in Milan and Copenhagen. I take part in the sales to clients who have been with the brand from the very beginning; other than that, it's taken care of by agents.

Does Copenhagen Fashion Week give you a good platform for international sales? In some ways it does. The show gives people around the world the chance to look at my work when they see the videos and runway pictures on the web and blogs. The sales are made in Paris during the Homme Fashion Week (almost all our buyers go to Paris), whereas Copenhagen is more of a media fashion week for us.

How do you prepare before your show? The best pieces often get created with the team the night before the show, but I prepare by creating a beautiful collection!

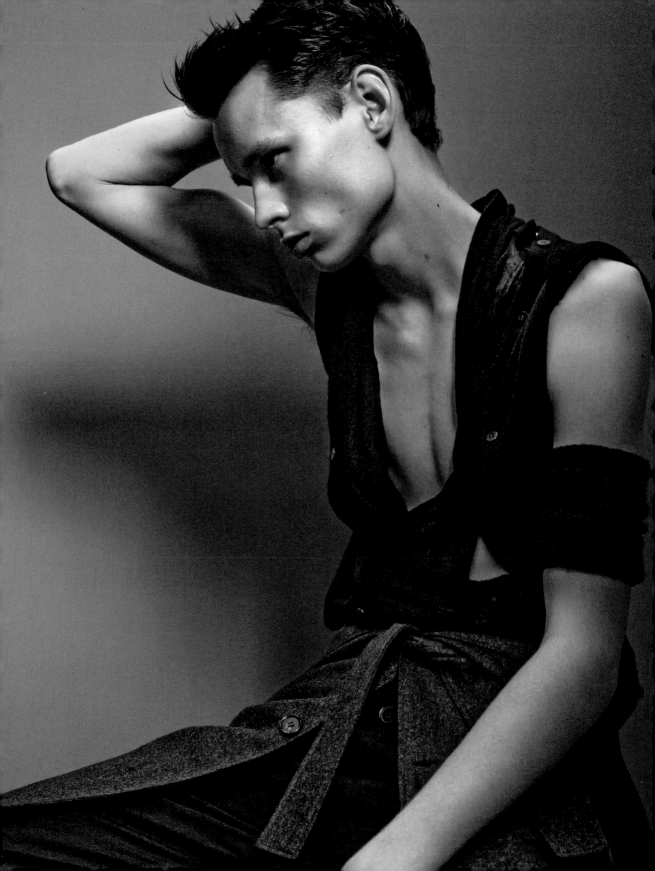

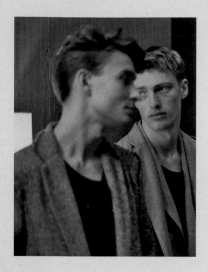

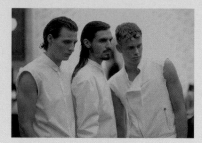

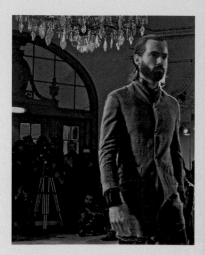

'The show gives people around
the world the chance to look
at my work when they see the
videos and runway pictures
on the web and blogs'

_____

ON FASHION WEEK

'I spent a lot of time by myself,
drawing and dreaming. I've
always been a loner, and still am'

_____

ON PERSONALITY

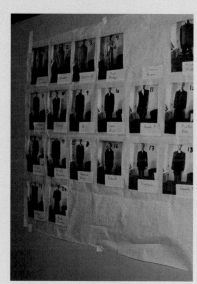

'If I set my mind to something,
I push until it gets to where
I want it to be, no matter
how it's created'

_____

ON DRIVE

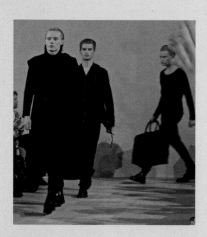

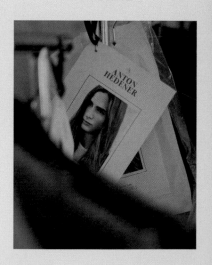

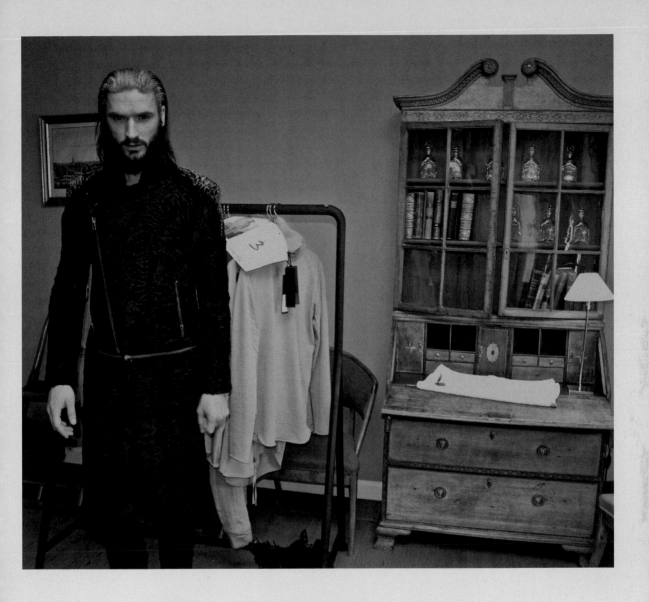

'The best pieces often get created with the
team the night before the show, but I prepare
by creating a beautiful collection'

_____

ON CREATIVITY

_____

JOHANNA PIHL

THIS INDEPENDENT SWEDISH TALENT HAS MANAGED TO RUN HER OWN
LABEL AFTER A LOT OF HARD WORK ON THE ROAD TO BECOMING A DESIGNER.
FROM HELPING WITH PRODUCTION TO STYLING AT THE WEEKENDS, SHE FINALLY
WENT TO ENGLAND TO STUDY WOMENSWEAR AT LONDON COLLEGE OF FASHION.
SEVERAL AWARDS LATER, SHE HAS DESIGNED FOR THE ENGLISH NATIONAL BALLET
AND HAD HER OWN SHOW DURING STOCKHOLM FASHION WEEK.

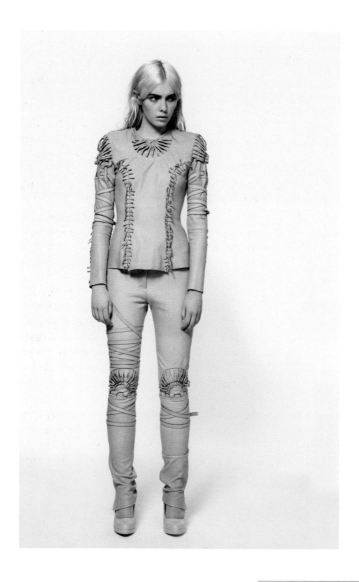

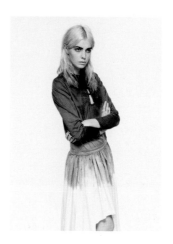

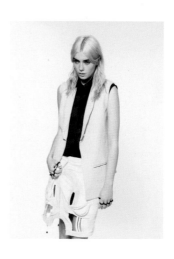

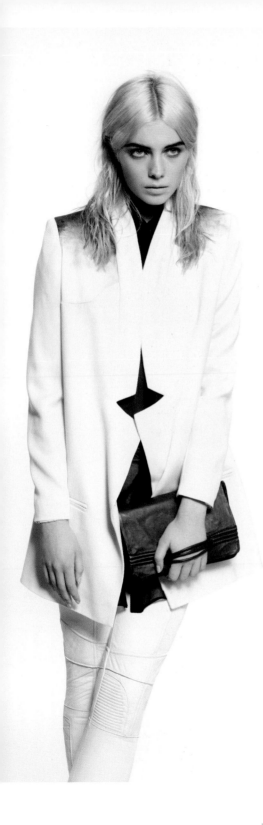

Your brand seems so fresh, with an international look. Tell me about your vision. When I design, I don't imagine a woman in a specific location because the woman I am designing for is everywhere in the world. I create clothes to highlight forward-thinking women in everyday life. I design with a strong, sharp and effortlessly stylish attitude for the woman who likes to reflect her inner style with her outer style.

Where did you start out, as regards education and work experience? From an early age I always had a great interest in clothes, and that interest was clarified by the women in my family, who also had a great passion for sewing and fashion. In order to shape my interest into something I could realize, I started to study sewing and pattern making, which led me on to a course in buying/production. After that I started working as a production manager at a clothing brand in Stockholm. That made me realize that I should follow what I always wanted to do, which was design, so I began to study art courses at night and work as a stylist's assistant at weekends. After a while I moved to London, where I did my BA in womenswear design at London College of Fashion. During those years while I studied, I also did work experience for different brands, and I think that is important for education as well.

What was your experience like, studying at London College of Fashion? I'm very glad that I studied in London. It's not only the city itself that's incredibly inspiring but also all the motivating people you meet. The education at London College of Fashion guided me to develop my own style and to believe strongly in what I create.

You did some styling experience as well, but did you decide that was not for you? When I worked as a stylist's assistant I thought it was great, and I really love the environment behind a shoot, but I felt all along that instead of being the one selecting the garments that were going to be photographed, I wanted to be the one who created the garments that were getting selected.

Are you inspired by anything or anyone when designing? Recurring interests I have are for architecture, interiors, objects and people I meet. But besides that, what I get inspired by changes constantly. It depends on what I feel passionate about, what I find new and interesting, and what I'm drawn to at the time.

When did you decide to start your own company, and why? It was always in my mind that I would like to start my

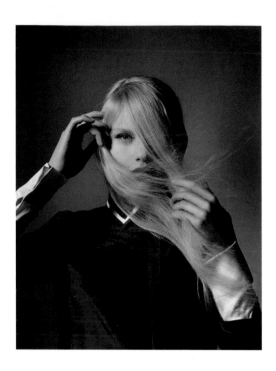

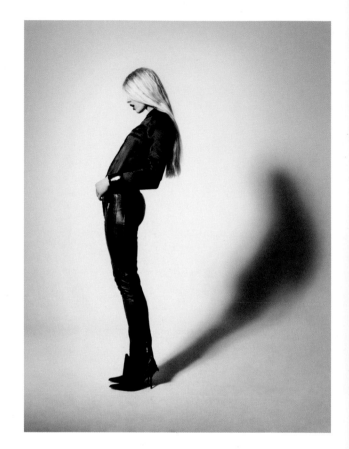

own business, and to my delight it went faster than I thought. When I finished my education in London in June 2011, I returned to Stockholm and took part in a competition sponsored by Mercedes-Benz – the Young Fashion Industry Award, which I won. The prize was that you got a show during Stockholm Fashion Week. This gave me the choice to continue working as an employee, which I was doing at the time, or to start my own label. It was then I felt it was the right time for me to start on my own, so I did.

You have won several competitions, including one to design for the English National Ballet. What makes your concepts strong? I always try to listen to my intuition and what feels right for me. I start by researching a lot, until I get completely absorbed in the concept I have built up, which gradually starts to form as my second world. For me it's important to be inspired by something I feel a great passion for, because I'm convinced that it will be reflected in the result.

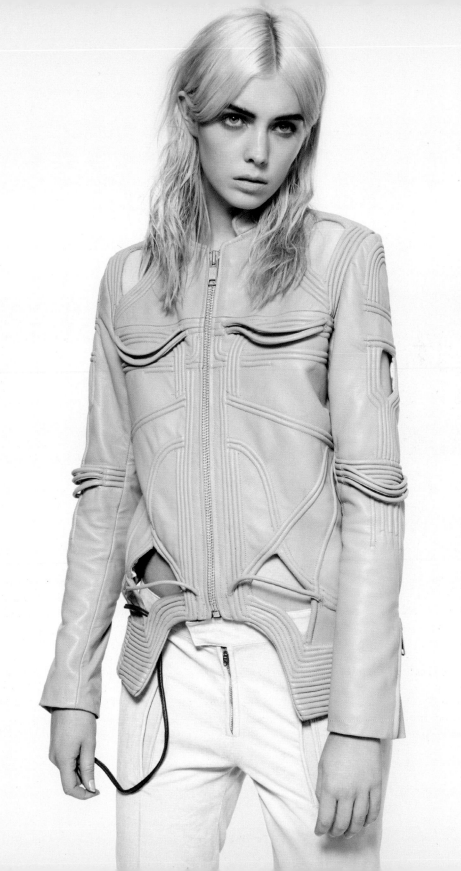

KALDA

ICELANDIC SISTERS KATRÍN ALDA AND REBEKKA RAFNSDÓTTIR STARTED THEIR
OWN BRAND IN 2010 AFTER RUNNING A SUCCESSFUL SHOP OF THE SAME NAME
IN REYKJAVIK. KATRÍN HAS A DEGREE IN FASHION, WHILE REBEKKA STUDIED PHILOSOPHY
AND CREATIVE WRITING. THE TWO COMBINE FORCES WITH A BRAND THAT
HAS ALREADY BEEN SOLD EXCLUSIVELY AT LIBERTY IN LONDON.

Katrín, can you describe what your brand is about?
It started when we opened our first shop in Reykjavik and then
we began to make our own clothes to sell there. It went really
well so we decided to establish an independent brand. We took
it slowly in the beginning and just made a few pieces of each
garment to find the road we wanted to take. We are now slowly
moving the business over to London.

**Are there any benefits for you as a company if you are
based in the UK?** There are a few reasons. Mainly I feel as if
I need to be surrounded by the best of the best to be able to
be competitive; 'in it to win it' kind of thing! Also there is no
support system in Iceland like there is in London. I got to know
the structure of the London fashion industry having studied
there for three years and then interned for a year afterwards.
I honestly think it's the best city for young designers to get the
support they need taking their first steps. Iceland obviously has
its pros, the most important for me being that it's very easy
to stimulate the imagination here, but in order to be able to
take the business further we need to surround ourselves with
industry knowledge, opportunities, support and competitors.

What are your backgrounds? I studied fashion management at London College of Fashion, and Rebekka studied
philosophy and creative writing at the University of Iceland.

**Which shops do you currently have your brand rep-
resented in?** About a year ago we presented our first full
womenswear collection and it was picked up exclusively by
Liberty in London. Apart from that we sell it in our own store
in Reykjavik.

**Amazing to be represented in Liberty! How did they
find out about you? Did they visit you in Iceland, or
do you show your collection during London Fashion
Week?** We were so, so happy when we got the deal. It meant
that we could take all the first steps to grow the business. We
showed the first collection at Copenhagen Fashion Week and
met the womenswear buyer from Liberty there.

**Your website and clothing look great – very New
Yorkish. I am surprised you are based in Iceland.**
Thanks! I guess it's a mix of both worlds. We're highly influenced by Iceland and its nature when we're creating, especially
when it comes to our prints, but at the same time we've always
seen the label as a global brand, so we're very aware of the
outside world.

**Do you get everything produced in Iceland, or how
do you manage? It must be expensive to ship…** We produced our first two collections entirely in Iceland but it turned
out to be too expensive for us. We've started working with
leather a lot so we need to source our fabric elsewhere. We're
currently testing out factories in India.

**Since you are two sisters doing the brand, I guess it
can be either a good thing or get very intense. How
is it to work with family in this way?** It's really good …
most of the time! You are able to be very honest and open with
each other so there's no underlying irritation, which is very
important when working so closely with someone.

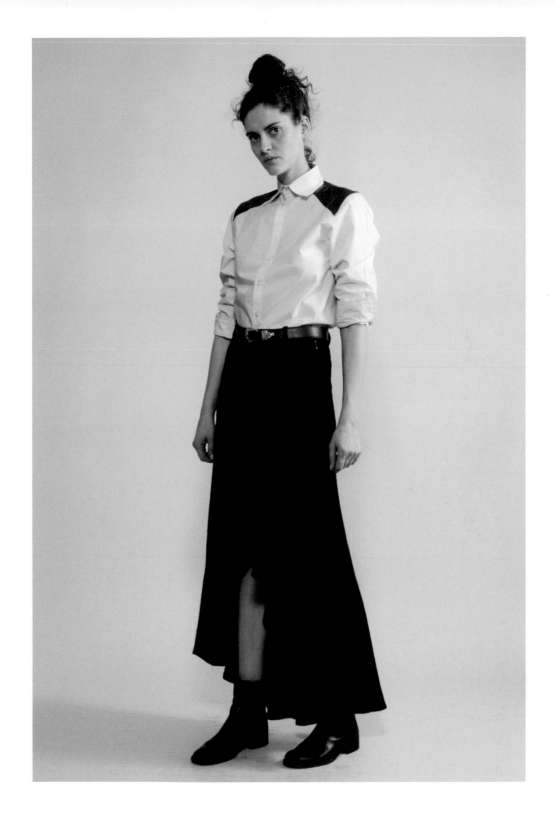

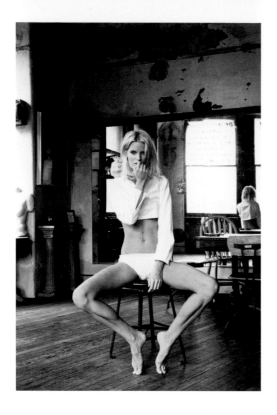

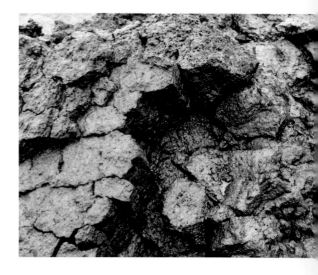

Above and below:
Icelandic landscape inspiration,
photographed by designer
Katrín Alda.

Below: Kalda collection
at Liberty in London.

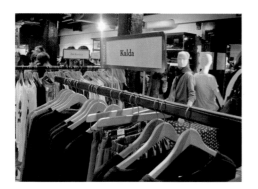

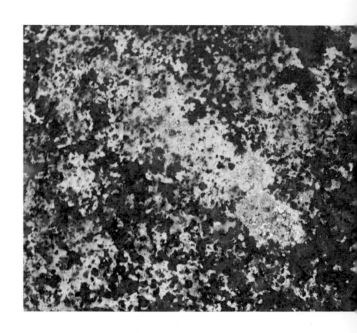

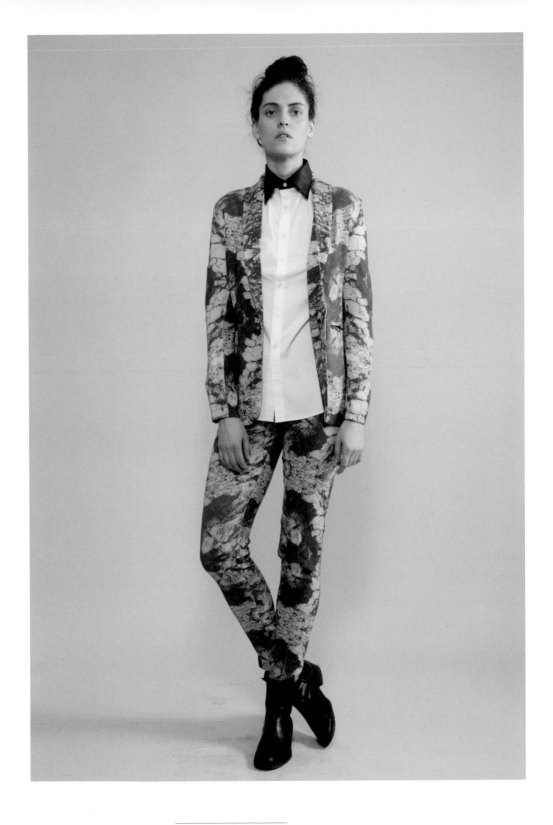

KRISTIAN AADNEVIK

THIS TALENTED DESIGNER IS BASED IN LONDON AND TAKES INSPIRATION FROM WELL-TRAVELLED INTERNATIONAL WOMEN MIXED WITH LANDSCAPE MEMORIES OF HIS NATIVE NORWAY. HE HAS A BACKGROUND AS A TAILOR, AN MA FROM THE ROYAL COLLEGE OF ART AND HAS WORKED FOR CHARLES JOURDAN. HE WAS ALSO CHOSEN BY DONATELLA VERSACE AS A 'PROTÉGÉ', WHICH MEANT HIS WORK WAS SEEN BY THE WORLD AT MILAN FASHION WEEK.

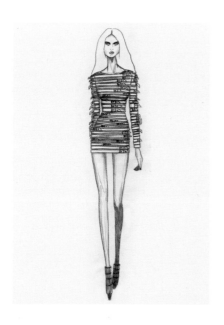

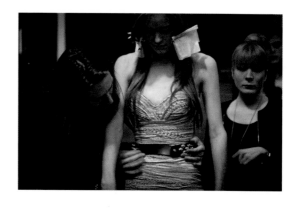

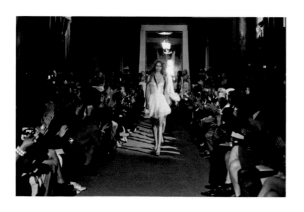

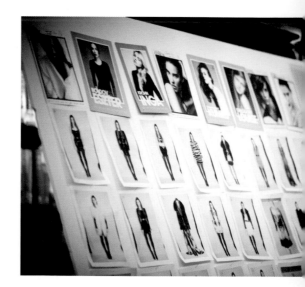

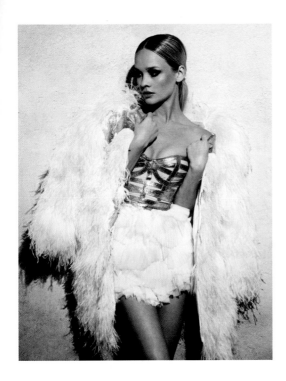

'For me, collections need
a story and emotions;
they're not just clothes'

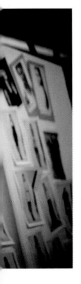

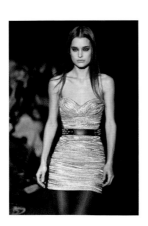

You were born in Norway, but are now based in London... Yes, I've been in London since 2000.

You graduated with an MA from the Royal College of Art. Where did you study before that? And I know the RCA is very intense, so how did you find the experience? Before RCA, I studied psychology at university and then I went on to a specialized tailoring academy in my hometown of Bergen. RCA was a great time and I developed a lot as a designer. What's so good about RCA is that not only is the fashion course very strong, but you also get to meet people from all the other creative courses, like product design, architecture, photography, fine art, etc. – all under the same roof. It's a very inspiring environment. RCA also has a fantastic network and they introduced me to the best fashion houses.

You have commented that your collections are like a film set. Are you inspired by any specific film maestros or genres? For me the collections need a story and emotions; they're not just clothes. Before I start each collection I always do lots of research and develop mood boards. You can start in one place and end up in another. It's a journey, and along the way pieces come together and become a story, very much like a film. My muse is the heroine. As a fashion designer, my creative mind is always open for inspiration, whether it's films, art, people or history.

Who is your heroine? My muse is in my imaginary world, but she is also a part of the many interesting women that I meet. She is fragile, mysterious and feminine, but also strong, ambitious and free. Her personality is of polarity – dark and light – and that is reflected through my style of mixing soft elements with hard: leather against chiffon and feathers against metal. She is independent and untamed and in the power of her own destiny.

Tell me about your time at Harrods and Charles Jourdan in Japan. Those were the first two companies I worked for, and I got the head design position for Harrods International straight from graduating. I was happy to have a well-paid job so quickly in this competitive industry. Both Harrods and Charles Jourdan were big collections, mainly for the Asian market. It was very good for me to design clothes that were all going into production and eventually into our own luxury stores. Japan, and especially Tokyo, is still one of my favourite destinations in the world for work and holiday.

Your dresses seem to appeal to a certain clientele – not very Scandinavian, more jetset. Is this a clear

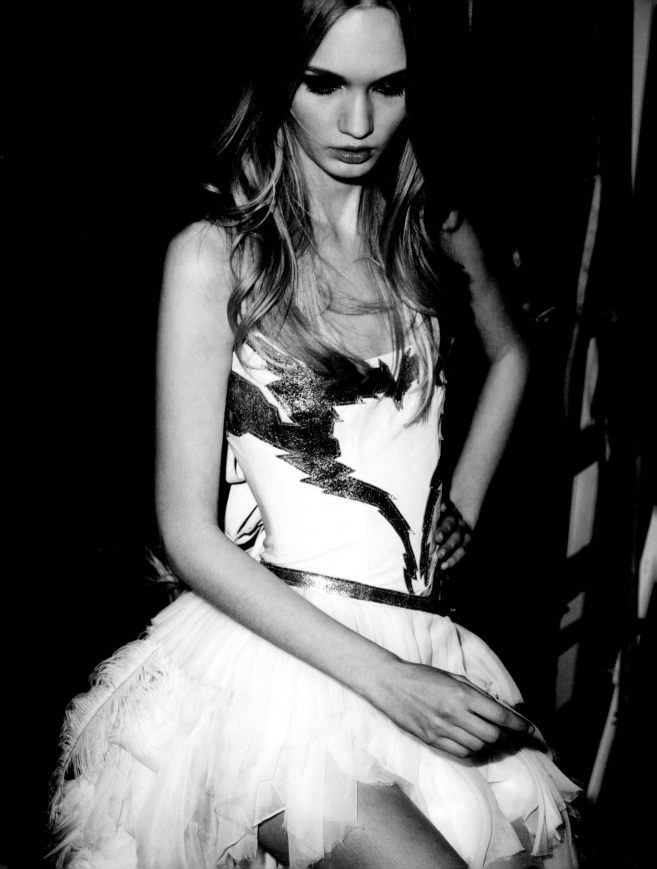

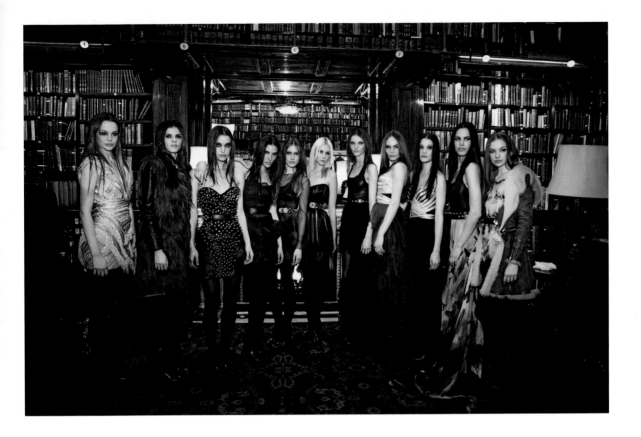

objective that you are designing for? I design with a creative vision that I believe in, and it's an evolving process. I think that it's for a very international woman, someone who travels a lot and lives life to the fullest. It's luxury fashion with a dark edge and a feminine shape.

Are you also working for Donatella Versace while designing for your own brand? I did a special project with Donatella when she selected me as her 'Versace Protégé'. It was an honour to be chosen and very inspiring to work together with her. The project culminated in a big gala show in Florence and eventually it went onto the runway for Milan Fashion Week.

Do you have any connection to Norway or are Scandinavian aesthetics in your mind when you design? There's often a dark edge to the collections I create. I find inspiration in Norse mythology, the dramatic nature of Norway, subcultures like Black Metal, and artists like Odd Nerdrum. The allure and sensuality is a longing…

Are all your dresses handmade and local? We make many of the more exclusive made-to-order pieces at the studio in London. Production is done in the UK, Italy and other places around the world.

Would you like to continue having your own brand or would you maybe design for someone else? To build my own brand is the main ambition and focus, but I'm also open to working for other fashion houses should the right opportunity arise one day.

KRISTOFER KONGSHAUG

THIS TALENTED YOUNG NORWEGIAN STUDIED AT THREE DIFFERENT
DESIGN SCHOOLS AND WORKED AT GIVENCHY AND ANNE VALÉRIE HASH
BEFORE STARTING HIS OWN COMPANY. HIS DEBUT COLLECTION WAS AWARDED
'COLLECTION OF THE YEAR' AT OSLO FASHION WEEK IN 2008. HE LIVES AT AND DESIGNS
FROM HIS STUDIO BASED IN PARIS AND PRESENTS TWO COLLECTIONS A YEAR,
WHILE A MEN'S LINE IS CURRENTLY IN DEVELOPMENT.

Tell me about the start of your brand. It started as a side project in 2007. Then in 2008 I got some more time – one and a half dedicated months, so not a lot of time, but some – and decided I might as well try. I was going to Norway on vacation, and Oslo Fashion Week was just around the corner. I contacted them and said I wanted to show, and they were happy to welcome me, so then I just had to stitch up the garments. It wasn't a very thought-through collection, as I managed to make it by myself in thirty days or less, and I probably could have edited it some more, but it was the first so I just went with it and it was just for fun. It went so well that I decided to continue the next season with a commercial collection, which I presented in my showroom in Paris.

How long have you been a designer now? It feels like forever, but I finished school in 2006.

You are based in Paris, aren't you? How come you wanted to move there, away from Norway? I left Norway in 2002. After a couple of years in Milan I went to Paris, where I finished school and started my first company with my partners, so when I started my own brand it was natural to stay in Paris, which has become my home.

Does Paris inspire the clothing that you want to make? Who knows? Paris is a heavy city. It takes a lot of energy from people. It's one of the most beautiful cities in the world but people never feel like it really belongs to them. Maybe that kind of sad atmosphere inspires me, and of course its rich history and tradition when it comes to tailoring. But as a team or idea, not really... All my work is about parallel life, emotion and shapes.

What is your technical background as a designer? I went to three different schools – Istituto Marangoni in Milan, ESMOD in Norway, then the Chambre Syndicale de la Haute Couture Parisienne. This has given me insight into how different schools can be and probably made me more open to doing things in many different ways. I don't really think your education matters. It's about the person, not the school. All you need is passion and practice in what you do. I love all sides of the business so I force myself to do them all, at least what I have time to, and that way I can master them.

Do you get your pieces produced abroad? Everything is produced in France and Italy.

What kind of fabrics do you use? I love natural fibres – wool, silk, ramie, etc. But I also use a lot of mixed fabrics and tech fabrics. Everything I make is based on cut and fabric.

I saw your show once in Norway and the models were bare-breasted. I commented in a Norwegian newspaper that I liked that you didn't care. Is part of being a designer for you making statements? Not really. What is a statement today? Everything has been done; nothing is shocking. I don't like showing too much skin, but I still love transparent fabrics. I love the female body – the shapes, the sensuality, the sexuality, all of it. It's the woman's choice what she wishes to expose. Transparency always leaves you the option to choose. You can always wear something underneath.

I recently used some of your pieces for _Vogue_ Italia and I loved the simple shapes but still how beautifully they were crafted. Do you do pattern cutting yourself,

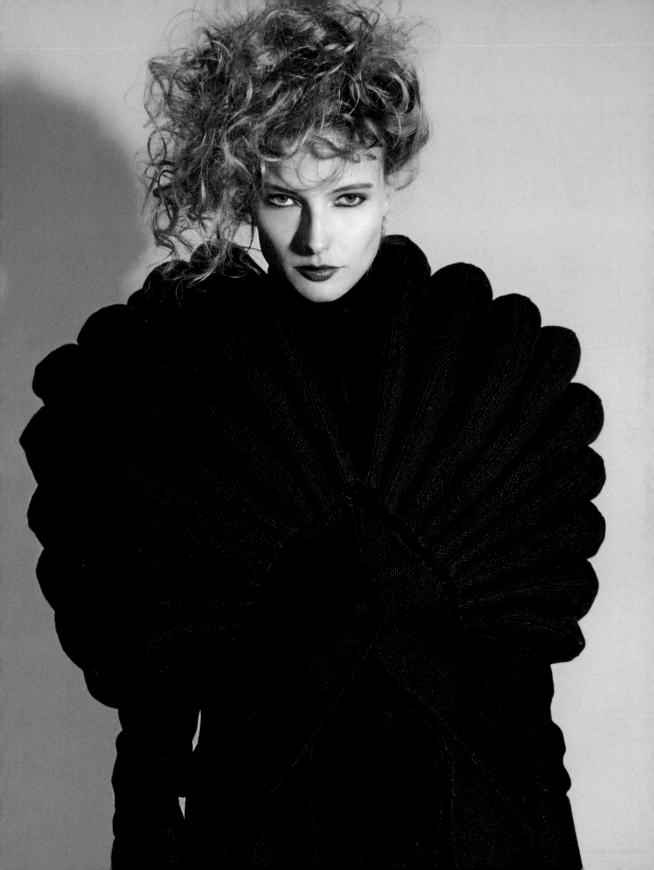

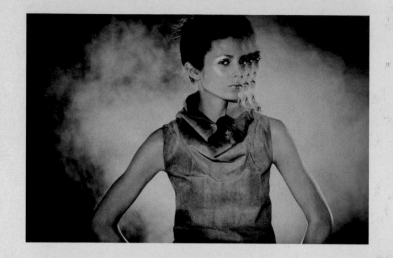

'I love the female body –
the shapes, the sensuality,
the sexuality, all of it'

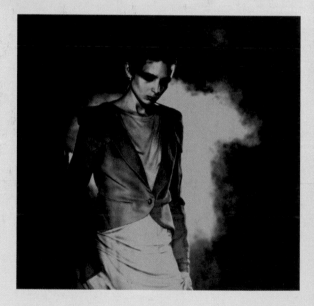

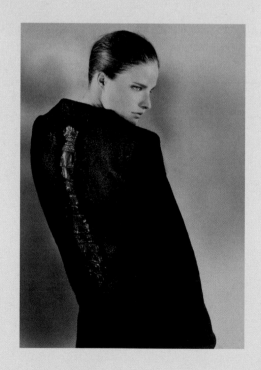

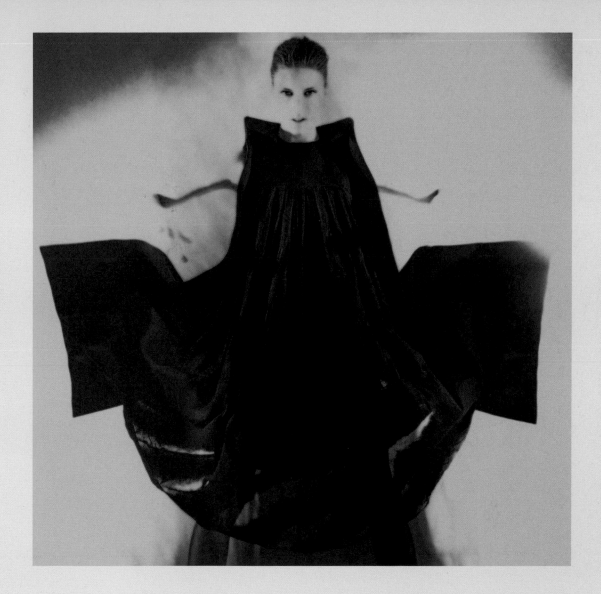

or do you have a little team? That's my passion. I do about 95% of all the patterns myself. Every garment in the collection is moulded on a doll (*moulage*). Then I have people who transform that into patterns, though sometimes I do it as well.

Who or what is your inspiration when you are designing? My little coven. Every collection is just a new chapter in the book. The inspiration changes with life, but the theme is the same.

Do you draw a lot, or is your process more technical? I do a lot of everything. It starts with a large amount of research and ideas, then sketches, then a selection, then a new selection, the *moulage* of the selection, then changes and so on. The most important part is the research and the *moulage*.

Where would you like to see your company going, or would you prefer to head a famous house? Who knows? One day at a time…

What is your next goal? Invasion! Ask me in a year's time. Maybe I will know then.

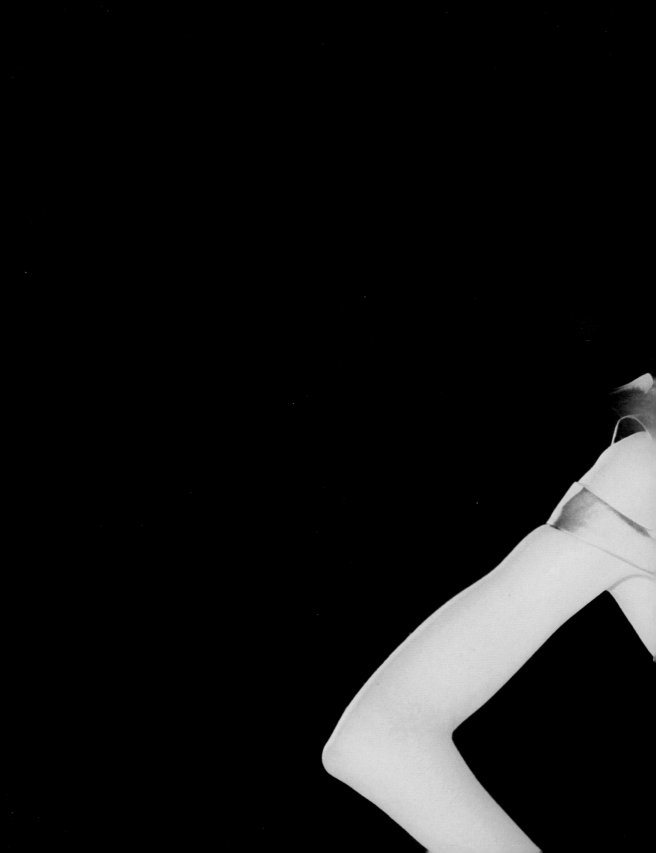

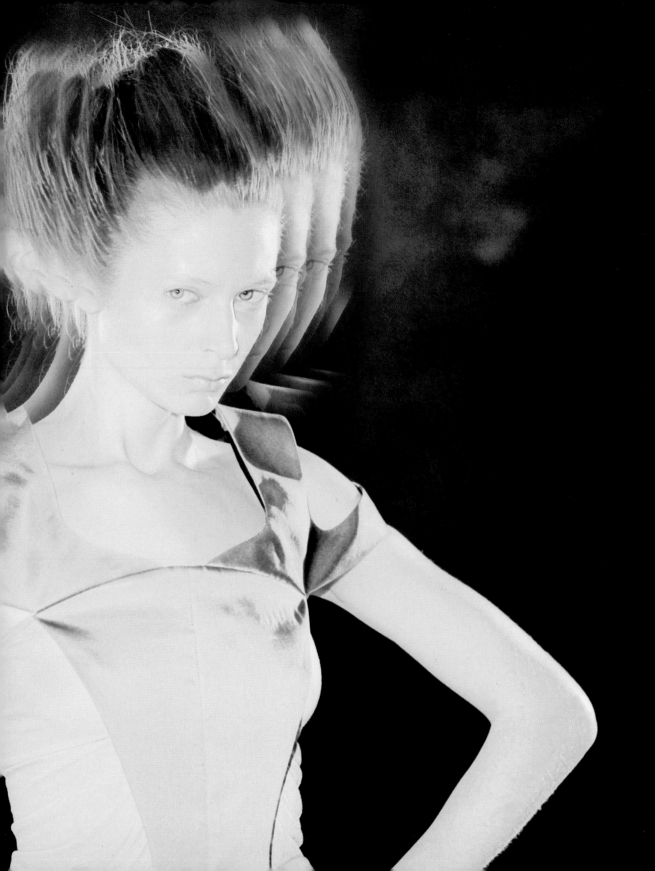

LIBERTINE-LIBERTINE

THREE CREATIVE SOULS – PERNILLE SCHWARZ, PETER OVESEN AND RASMUS BAK –
CREATED THIS DYNAMIC DANISH BRAND, WHICH NOW HAS RETAILERS WORLDWIDE.
THEY PRESENT THEIR COLLECTION IN LOCATIONS RANGING FROM NEW YORK TO PARIS,
WHILE LIVING LIKE HOBOS AND TAKING INSPIRATION FROM THE SURFING
COMMUNITY AND OTHER FREE-MINDED SPIRITS.

Rasmus, how did you three start out in fashion?
Pernille has a Masters from Kolding School of Design and has been designing collections since graduating in 2004, Peter studied philosophy and creative business, and I have a vast background within music, fashion and other creative fields. Though our backgrounds are very different, and our meeting in the first place was coincidental, we've all found the fashion business to be the perfect platform for realizing creative initiatives and amazing product development.

Tell me about the idea behind the brand and the name. Libertine-Libertine was founded in the summer of 2009 with the ambition of launching a brand based on a different set of business values, fresh energy and collections of excellent quality and craftsmanship. Simultaneously we wanted to build a versatile platform that allowed us to engage in different cultural activities that we feel connected to and that have inspired us throughout the years – bright cities and wild shores. The name Libertine-Libertine was born during a stay in Paris and refers to our sense of independence and freedom, both of which are highly regarded in every corner of our business.

What was it like starting your own company? It's been an incredible adventure. We started out with a collection of fifteen pieces because that was all we could afford to do. The recession was still on everybody's lips and borrowing even €1,000 was impossible. However, it taught us great will and stubbornness in terms of making this real and focusing on the content, the journey and doing things right. It was – and still is – incredibly hard work, which requires absolute dedication and the ability to navigate in the chaotic scenery that is the fashion industry. We are still enjoying the ride and the huge progress we have made in quite a short amount of time, and I wouldn't trade the long nights and thousands of miles in the car for anything.

Is your collection designed, manufactured and produced in Denmark? That is unfortunately not possible. We have neither the facilities in the country nor the financial option to do so. However, we keep all our production in Europe, mainly in Italy, Portugal and Turkey. We have a very high production standard and want to keep our partners close, almost local.

Were you based in a country other than Denmark at one point? Our HQ has always been in Copenhagen but the past two years have been spent constantly travelling to key cities in the world. We embrace this hobo way of life and in many ways it unconsciously brings a lot of good energy back to the brand.

You present your collection at 'Capsule' in New York and Paris. Do you find this a good platform for sales and new designers? We exhibit in Paris, Berlin, New York and Copenhagen, as well as in various showrooms around Europe. The two shows you mention have been great platforms, but a lot of preparation is required prior to exhibiting.

You seem to be very popular in England. Is this a market that reminds you of Scandinavia? The UK has been a strong market for us since the very first collection. Both retailers and consumers get our brand mentality and appreciate the quality and detailing in the collections. It's always a pleasure with the Brits and there is cohesion in some cardinal points of life and culture, but it doesn't remind me much of Scandinavia.

Will you be working on any collaborations in the near future? We have loads of new projects in the pipeline, which will be revealed when the time is right. Keep track online!

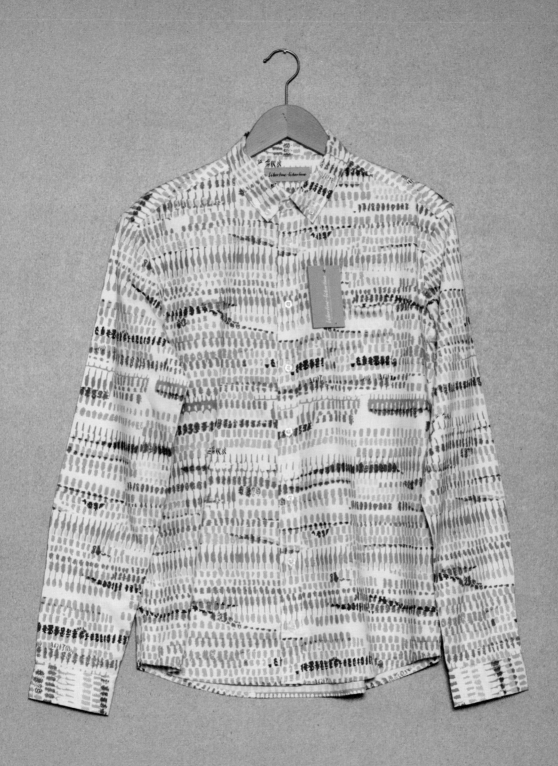

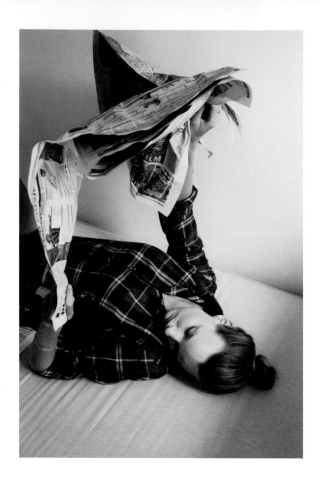

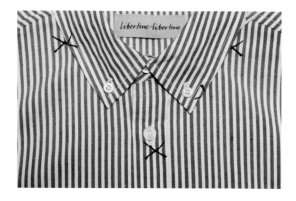

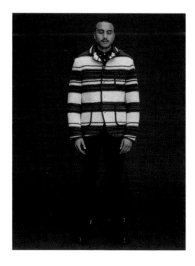

Above right: Shirt collaboration with surf brand Oh Dawn.

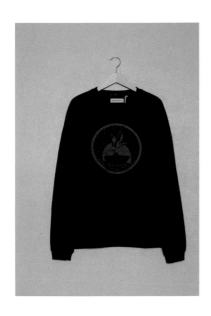

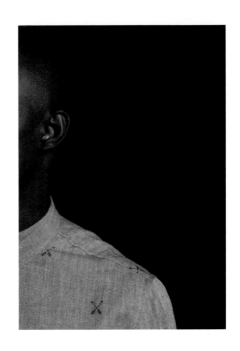

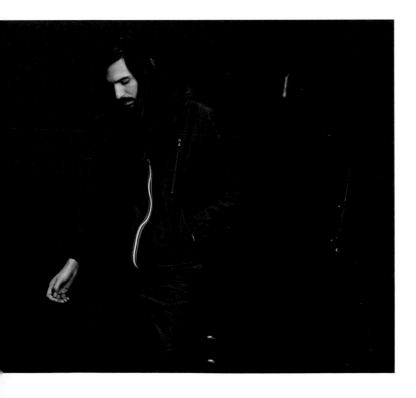

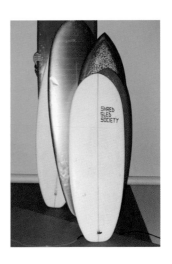

LOUISE SIGVARDT

FRESH ON THE DANISH FASHION SCENE IS THIS TALENTED DESIGNER,
WHO RECENTLY GRADUATED FROM KOLDING SCHOOL OF DESIGN. SHE WAS
HEADHUNTED TO WORK AT BRUUNS BAZAAR EVEN BEFORE SHE HAD WON THE TOP
SCANDINAVIAN DESIGN PRIZE, 'DESIGNER'S NEST', JUDGED BY THE LIKES OF SARA
MAINO AT VOGUE ITALIA AND HILARY ALEXANDER AT THE DAILY TELEGRAPH.

Tell me about being a new designer today. First of all, I've been most fortunate in my brief career, having worked with some of the best from the Copenhagen fashion scene and having had the opportunity to create a new collection after my graduation collection during my work at a large fashion brand. But I think the time now is for creative designers, because the fashion industry needs to think outside the box. It's not enough to find the most expensive materials poured over a classic shape. To stand out, designers must experiment with the whole range.

You graduated from Kolding School of Design. What was it like studying there? Since it's quite remote, I'm wondering what you did in your spare time… A lot of people have asked me that question, and the question almost answers itself because, when you don't have a lot of options in your spare time, you tend to spend all of your time at school. The combination of too much time and dedicated students adds up to a massive amount of good energy and the possibility of always having someone to talk to about your design. And those sparring parters have turned out to be a strong part of my network. Kolding is a great school in many ways: one reason is because the location is remote, so you tend to be less inspired by local influences and are thus forced either to develop your own expression or to seek inspiration from a more global perspective. Also the main staff is very limited so most of the teachers are externals and new, innovative designers, who all have different perspectives on design, which means that you have a lot of options when choosing your design style.

You won the 'Designer's Nest' competition in 2012, judged by _Vogue_ Italia and Hilary Alexander. Tell me about that experience. At first I seriously considered staying at home because I didn't think I'd win, but when I got there I met up with some classmates from school, standing in the back drinking free drinks. When it got to the announcements and they called my name as the winner, it was completely surreal. So from when they called my name to the end of the day is still kind of a haze. I only really remember saying thank you a lot to the Crown Princess of Denmark. But the best part was the statements from the judges recorded for Copenhagen Fashion Week.

Do you start from scratch every time you design a new collection? My main inspiration for each collection is unique. I spend a lot of time developing the theme and the story behind the clothes – before even drawing a sketch – but some of the cuts and details can easily be developments from a previous collection, or details that were made before but didn't suit the previous collection and now fit the new one better.

Do you make everything by hand? How do you proceed? I like to call my process a 'non-linear' process, in which I don't have one straight line of work or one specific sketch medium. I tend to move back and forth during the process and, depending on the collection, use different sketch methods, such as paper cutouts with added coloured pencil. Another process was when I chose neoprene as the main fabric and used the material itself to get a feel for what was possible and what would work aesthetically.

Where are your fabrics and materials from? Before beginning my graduation collection, I took an inspiration trip to Tokyo, where I found some very special Japanese polyester and denim fabrics that later became the basis of the collection.

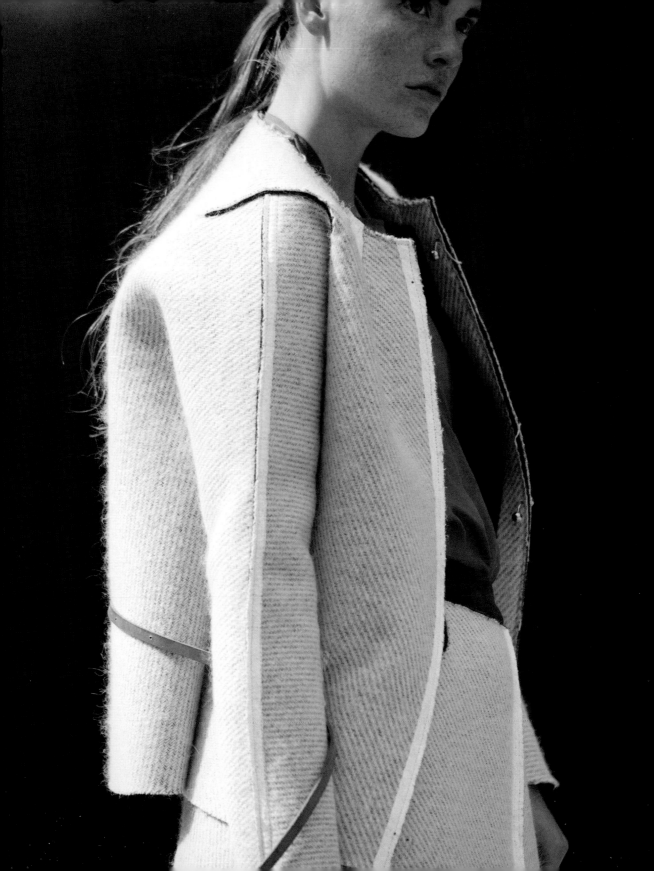

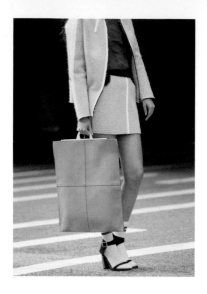

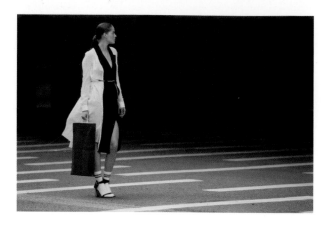

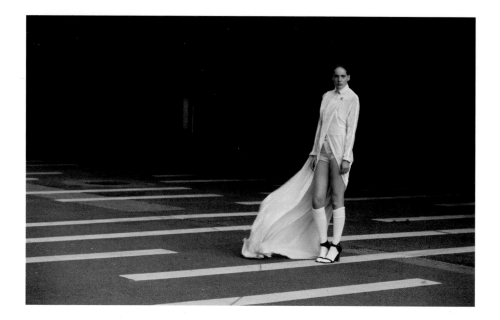

Where do you sell your collection? For my graduation collection and my first professional collection, all the pieces were handmade to measure as one-offs and only sold on request. It was actually never the purpose of the collection to be the start of a fashion brand, but a PR studio offered to manage the collection and said that if anyone was interested it would be possible to buy the pieces through them.

What has been going on since you won? What are you planning on now? After winning 'Designer's Nest', I was featured in numerous Danish magazines. The title has been a very good stamp of approval for my future career. But just before I won I was hired by Bruuns Bazaar [see p. 42], who have recently changed their design strategy, so all in all I think the most exciting work is in Denmark right now.

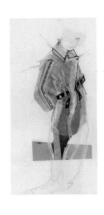

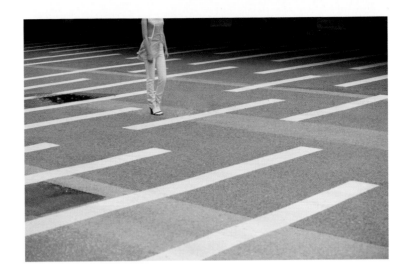

'I think the time now is for creative designers, because the fashion industry needs to think outside the box'

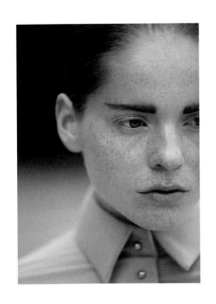

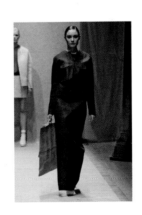

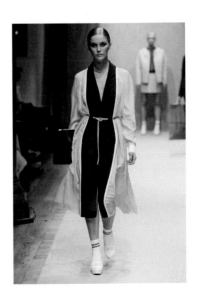

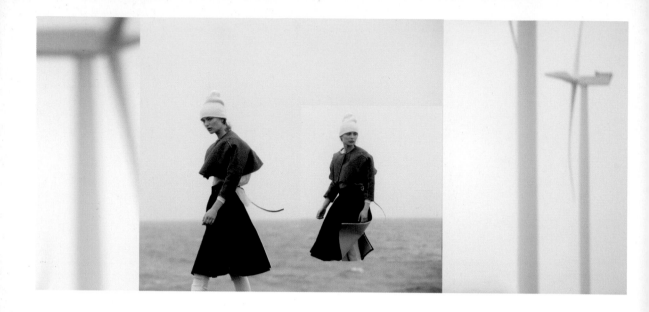

'I spend a lot of time
developing the theme and
the story behind the clothes –
before even drawing a sketch'

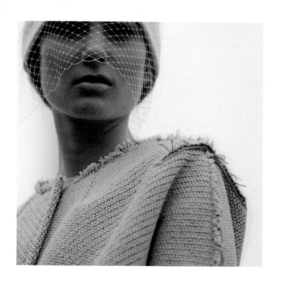

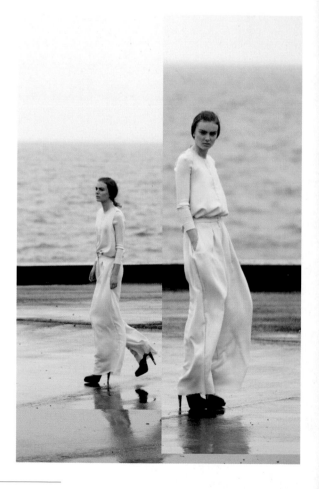

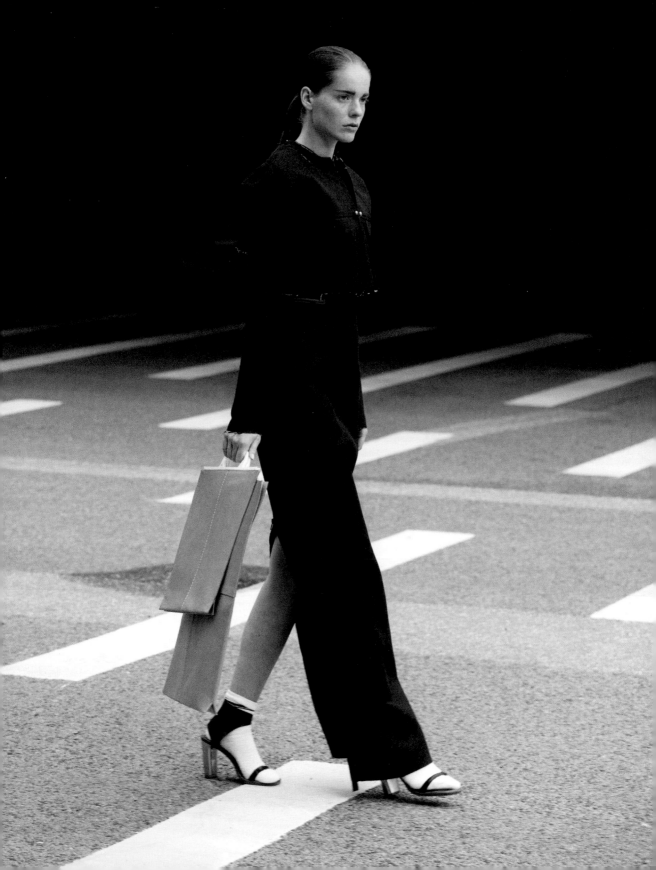

MARIA NORDSTRÖM

THIS NEW SWEDISH DESIGNER FEATURED AT STOCKHOLM FASHION WEEK AND QUICKLY BECAME A FIRM FAVOURITE. IT WAS AFTER A STINT AT H&M THAT SHE REALIZED SHE WANTED TO CREATE PIECES THAT LOOKED AS BEAUTIFUL ON THE INSIDE AS ON THE OUTSIDE. SHE IS A CONFIDENT FIGHTER WHO LOVED PERFORMING WITH HER BAND BUT NOW DECLARES HER TAILORED CLOTHING TO BE HER ART FORM.

I saw your collection for the first time during Stockholm Fashion Week in January 2012. I was very impressed by your graphic garments with beautiful backs. To me you are like a Scandinavian Rick Owens-meets-Haider Ackermann. Tell me about your background. I was born on the west coast of Sweden, in Gothenburg. As a child I was extremely impressed by my three older sisters and the art/grunge air around their lifestyle. I grew up in a neighbourhood full of brats, but I dressed myself in vintage clothing and pieces I stitched together the best I could. To wear an old scarf safety-pinned into a dress, together with a big green hat, was nothing weird to me, and I styled everything with my yellow Docs. So when I started doing fashion I hadn't got much knowledge of how a garment 'should' look. And in school I did my best to push the boundaries of design. Therefore it was very different to start working for H&M. I had to make a shirt look like a proper shirt, with all the details in the right place. When I left, something had changed. I suddenly wanted to do more of a hybrid of fashion. When I first started my label in 2009, I was filled with the idea that I wanted to make fashion my way, not compromise my designs in any way. I had also just left my band Zeigeist, which had been a great creative output for me.

How did you have time to do fashion and music? The two are of course intertwined, but fashion can take so much time … as can rehearsing! But then again it's all a creative output. Zeigeist was a passion project of mine for many years and I think that the way we worked together – five artists from five different scenes, trying to create a new kind of performance – made me flexible and used to working with all kinds of media (we did everything together, from set design to film, which always changed for every gig). Somewhere along the way it became my way of hanging out with friends and talking about and making new projects … which also applies to how I do things now with the awesome people I surround myself with at work.

Do you feel that fashion is your visual version of the music you make? The total opposite actually. Zeigeist had a very direct way of expressing itself. My collections, on the other hand, have been worked through carefully – every cut, every shade and material cautiously nursed to perfection. And I love it. Since the garments are not a part of me, as my singing and performing were, I can adjust and change them into whatever I want them to be. There are no boundaries.

You seem to have a couture feel in your clothes. Have you ever worked in that field or anything similar? I was heading in that direction for a long time, and I have chosen to work with elements of couture-making. The materials and manufacture are always of the finest quality: the insides are almost as beautiful as the outsides. But the appearance is in between high fashion and couture. There's couture craftsmanship and the expression of straightforward fashion, since I think fashion needs to encapsulate a feeling of its present time. That's one aspect of what makes it so interesting. My other big passion is based on the idea of garments interacting with personality – the way both the wearer and the clothing transform when their personae are perfectly intertwined.

You say that you combine fashion with art and that you do not differentiate. Why do you think it is so hard for people to accept that some fashion can actually be a wearable form of art? Art is excluding, exclusive, for some people. Whether you like it or not, fashion is something

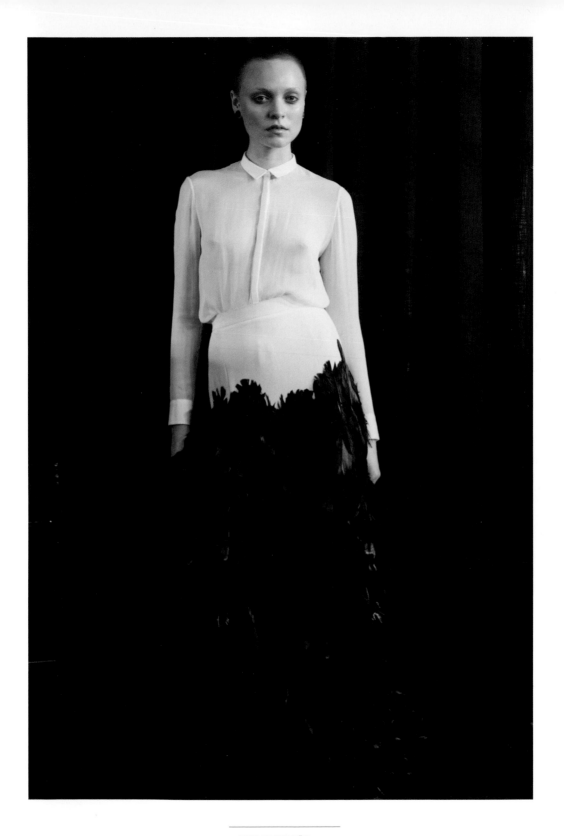

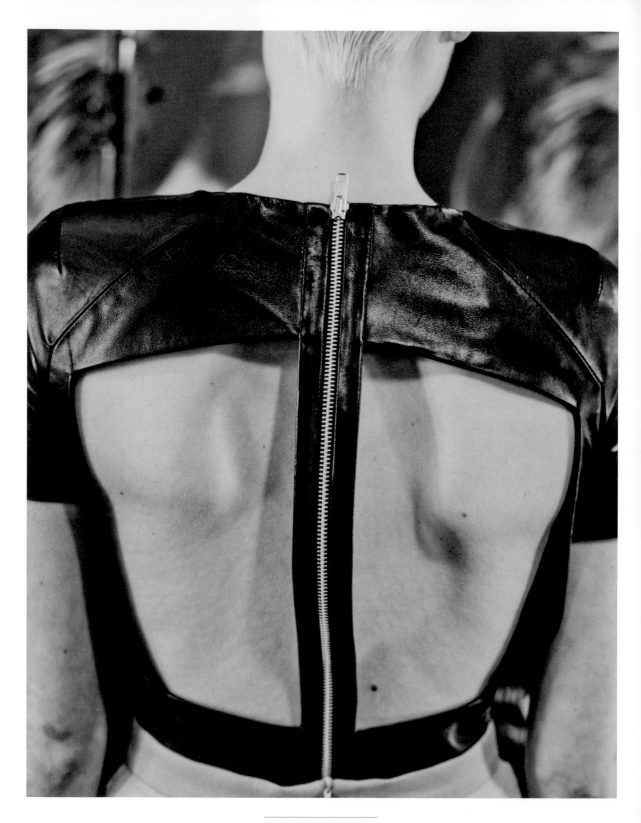

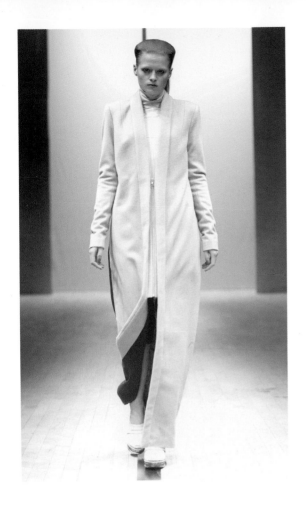

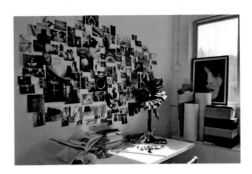

Above: The atelier in Stockholm.

Below: A seashell detail from a showpiece jacket.

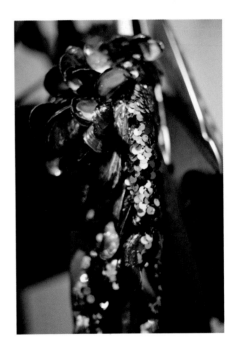

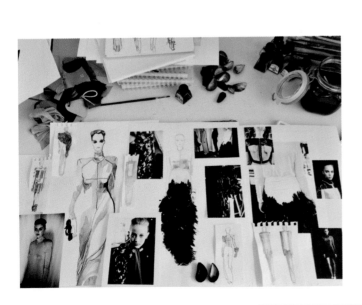

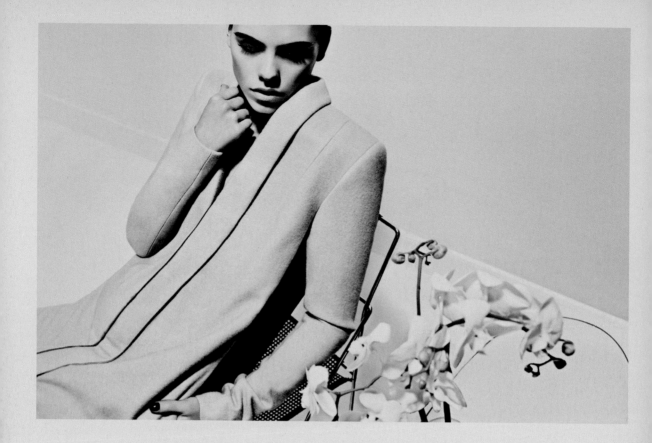

everyone has to have an opinion on, since we all wear clothes. I would guess that the people who don't understand a more complex beauty – far from sunsets and kittens – are the ones who are profoundly offended that anyone would go so far as to call pieces of cloth put together to keep you warm 'Art'.

Where does your inspiration come from for your collections? The '01 Purgatory' collection was about Catholic ambivalence – the conflict between sin and virtue, dressed and stripped, calm and aggressive. This, I must add, was a completely visual inspiration for the collection; I myself have very few ties to religion. I tried to visualize the paradigm of asceticism from a modern fashion perspective.

Where do you work from? What is your studio like? Is it crammed with inspiration, or clean and simple? How do you prefer to work? I work in three phases, one

might say. My home is my sanctuary for sketching and inspiration. In my studio I keep all the equipment I need, and the place is completely crowded with machines, dummies, fabric and so on (that is where I make the first try-outs and toiles of new ideas). And finally, in my tailor's studio, she and I work together to complete the garments.

To make a brand that is fashion-meets-art must be difficult financially. Do you get funding? How do you manage to produce your collections? If there's a will there's a way.

Tell me what would happen in the future with your brand if you could decide. I would continue to make collections in the same spirit and let the label grow organically. Right now we are looking for new ways to produce in Europe and for stores that fit the brand.

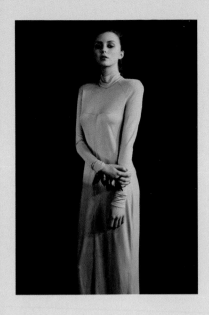

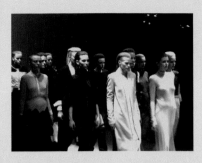

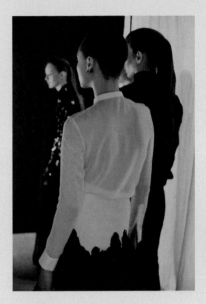

'The materials and manufacture
are always of the finest quality:
the insides are almost as
beautiful as the outsides'

ON DESIGN

'When I first started my label,
I was filled with the idea that I
wanted to make fashion my way,
not compromise my designs'

ON DRIVE

'A big passion is based on the
idea of garments interacting
with personality – the way both
wearer and clothing transform
when their personae are
perfectly intertwined'

ON PERSONALITY

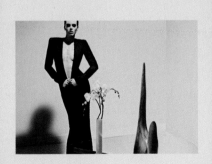

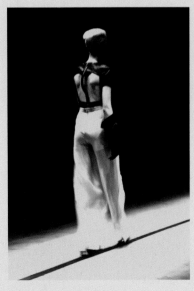

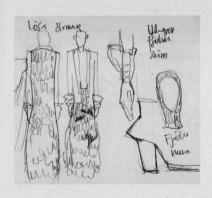

MARIMEKKO

ONE OF SCANDINAVIA'S MOST RENOWED BRANDS, WITH DESIGNS EMBRACED BY THE LIKES OF JACKIE KENNEDY AND 'SEX IN THE CITY' STYLIST PATRICIA FIELDS, THIS COMPANY TAKES GOOD CARE OF THE ENVIRONMENT AND SETS A PERFECT EXAMPLE BY PRODUCING ALL ITS PRODUCTS IN FINLAND, THEREBY ALSO CREATING JOBS AND RECYCLING MATERIALS. THE CREATIVE DIRECTOR IS MINNA KEMELL-KUTVONEN.

Minna, tell me about the beginning of Marimekko.
Armi Ratia and her husband Viljo launched Marimekko in 1951. Finland was getting back on its feet after World War II and people were longing for bright colours and fresh ideas. Armed with only a dream of a world in which beauty and practicality were inseparable, Armi was fearless. She set about transforming her husband's textile company, Printex, into a living dream and was one of the first to gather up-and-coming artists and commission them to create fresh and radical designs.

You employ a large number of designers. Does each come with their own style, which is adapted to the Marimekko universe? How do they work together?
At Marimekko we give our designers creative freedom. They are committed to timelessness, in terms of both long-lastingness and visual timelessness. As the founder Armi Ratia said: 'Marimekko is not about trendy fashion. We make timeless and lasting products, which are by chance often very fashionable.' We work with around 20–25 designers, both renowned Marimekko masters as well as young design talents growing in-house to become the Marimekko masters of tomorrow.

You have had different designers setting the tone over time but always kept the recognizable patterns, such as the Poppy. What has inspired the design most?
There's a nice story behind that print. Armi Ratia had publicly forbidden all Marimekko designers from creating floral prints, because she felt that flowers would always be much more beautiful in nature. However, designer Maija Isola didn't care about restrictions and went ahead and designed a whole series of plant- and floral-inspired prints, one of them being 'Unikko'. She showed the design to Armi, who changed her mind, as 'Unikko' was not a traditional floral print. And there

it has been ever since and has become the most iconic design of our design house!

Jackie Kennedy famously wore Marimekko. How did she get hold of it back then? We know Jacqueline Kennedy bought nine Marimekko cotton dresses in 1960 during the presidential election campaign. She wore one of them on the cover of *Sports Illustrated* magazine. In 2011 – to celebrate our 60th anniversary – we brought that dress model, designed by Vuokko Eskolin-Nurmesniemi, back into production. The fact that Jackie wore our dresses was very daring at the time and still inspires us and the friends of Marimekko alike.

You seem to have a great factory in Sulkava by the lakeside. Is the company solely based in Finland for production, or elsewhere too? We've decided to develop profitable manufacturing in our home country and we are very proud of our three company-owned factories. Our textile printing factory, in connection with our headquarters in Helsinki, prints most of our fabrics – around 1.5 million metres a year. In 2011 we invested in a new printing machine, which tripled Marimekko's textile printing factory's output capacity. The overall trend in the sector is completely different, but we want to go against the trend because we believe that being a pioneer in pattern design goes hand-in-hand with in-house production. Our bag factory in Sulkava makes our classic bags. Purses and tricot clothes are sewn in Kitee.

Marimekko has had its ups and downs since the 1960s, then it was used in a *Sex and the City* episode by stylist Patricia Fields and became popular once again. What do you think has made customers return?
Marimekko has boldly walked its own path since the beginning.

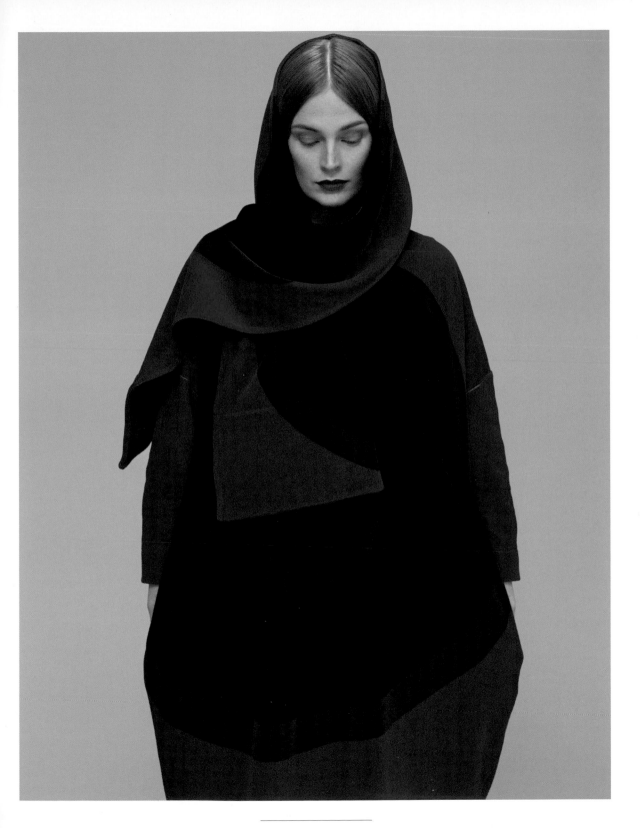

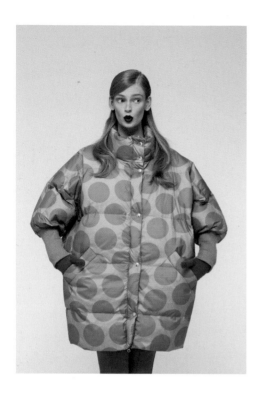

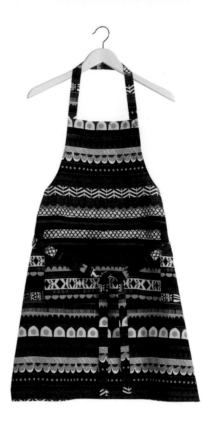

It has remained true to its philosophy of bold colours and patterns. One of the reasons we feel that it is more topical today than ever before is due to the shift in people's values, kick-started by the financial crisis. This has led many consumers to shift from status-symbol brands to brands that have perhaps more personality and radiate authenticity. Rather than dressing themselves in a brand, consumers are looking for their own individual style – they may even mix brands from very different price-points – and through that they communicate who they are.

You are very aware of your corporate responsibilities, such as using fabrics that guarantee ecological sustainability. You don't have much waste either, and do things like make purses from cut-offs. All in all you don't seem to hide any nasty details of production or low quality. Can you tell me about your vision with this side of the company? When we design, a lot of effort is made to figure out the environmental impact of materials, and recyclability as well as lifecycle issues. Durability has become one of the chief benchmarks of a product's ecological acceptability. We firmly believe that a well-designed, timeless,

high-quality and functional product will bring joy to its user for a long time: it won't be abandoned when fashion shifts. Ideally, this fondness will last from generation to generation, from mother to daughter, even granddaughter. Also, taking care of our products correctly is highlighted by our store personnel. This is very important because as much as two-thirds of the emissions and energy consumption during a textile product's lifecycle comes from washing and maintenance after the actual manufacturing. We avoid overpacking and we aim to make packaging materials recyclable. The company also aims to improve the management of its whole order/delivery chain and to further increase the transparency of its supply chain through, for example, membership in the Business Social Compliance Initiative.

Tell me about a typical day at the Marimekko office.
I don't think there really is a typical day at Marimekko! Our days here are full of energy, working together with people from different parts of the design house – overall about being creative, no matter what we do. It's a lot of fun to work in the 'Marimekko family'!

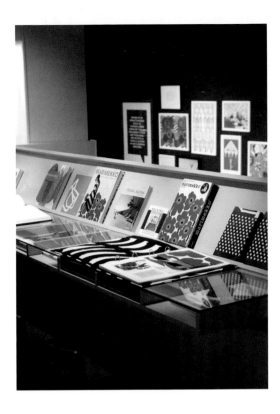

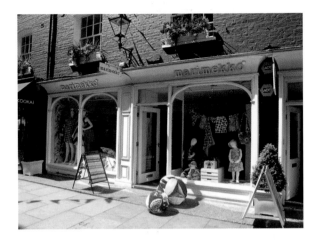

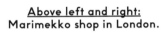

<u>Above left and right:</u>
Marimekko shop in London.

<u>Below:</u> A Marimekko
factory in Finland.

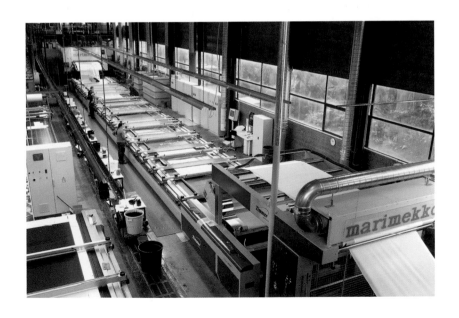

MINIMARKET

THREE SISTERS – SOFIE, PERNILLA AND JENNIFER ELVESTEDT – ARE BEHIND ONE OF SWEDEN'S MOST POPULAR DESIGNER BRANDS, WELL KNOWN FOR ITS USE OF COLOUR AND PRINT. THE SISTERS SHOWCASE THEIR COLLECTIONS IN COPENHAGEN AND STOCKHOLM, AND DESIGN A COLLECTION EVERY SEASON WITH 'PRICE OPENERS' THAT SHARE HIGH QUALITY BUT AT A LOWER COST. NEXT WE MIGHT SEE MENSWEAR OR EVEN BABYWEAR ON THE SHELVES.

Tell me a bit about the beginning of Minimarket and why you created it. We ran a store and started making pieces ourselves when we couldn't find everything we needed from our featured designers. Our own pieces sold very quickly, so we closed the shop and focused on design and production.

You are three sisters. Tell me about each of your roles in the company. We used to design everything together, but now we have developed our roles into Sofie handling the strategics of the collection and prints, while Pernilla and Jennifer focus on drawing the garments and shoes.

In an interview I once did with you, you commented that in your collection you are developing a 'price opener', so that younger people can afford to buy it. Tell me about this. Each 'chapter' (jackets, shoes, etc.) is built with a range of prices, based on how advanced the pattern construction is and what material we use. Our own prints are of course always more expensive to produce, while a black cupro is more affordable. We want each price range to start at an affordable level, and therefore we always have a look at our different options to fulfill this.

If you produce cheaper garments for a younger audience, do you get them produced in a different place from the rest of your collection? No, everything is produced in the same factories. We tried making cheaper products in cheaper factories, but it is very hard to achieve our specified level of quality and ethics when the production price is lower than a certain point, so we have included these products in our regular range with our regular suppliers. Usually the 'price openers' are high-quantity pieces, which in itself motivates the lowered production price.

When you began your brand, did you work on it full-time or did you have jobs on the side to manage the costly start-up of a company? In the beginning, Pernilla and Jennifer worked with care of the elderly and Sofie did some freelance copywriting work.

What are you inspired by? Usually characters and phenomena – myths as well as historical facts. We worked with Shangri-La as the inspiration for our SS13 collection.

Are you based in Stockholm full-time? If so, why do you showcase in Copenhagen? Is it to have a larger platform? We are based in Stockholm, but we absolutely love Copenhagen. Nowadays, we show every other season in Stockholm and every other season in Copenhagen in order to entertain both cities. Copenhagen is more relaxed than Stockholm, but also more interested in fashion. In Stockholm, only fashion people and a few other interested people know when it is Fashion Week; in Copenhagen everybody knows. Also Copenhagen has always welcomed us with open arms and that has been hard to resist. Stockholm is our hometown, however, and we are so happy that the Swedish audience is finally daring to wear colours and prints.

Sofie, where do you want to take the brand? What are your wishes for the future? At the moment we are focusing on Scandinavia. We are also starting up a collaboration with one of our favourite Japanese distributors. Further on, we will have to start a menswear line, as we have so many requests for that. Having just become a mother, I of course am also very keen to start up a kidswear section! But, realistically, I would say the menswear and a few of our own shops will be reality before the babywear.

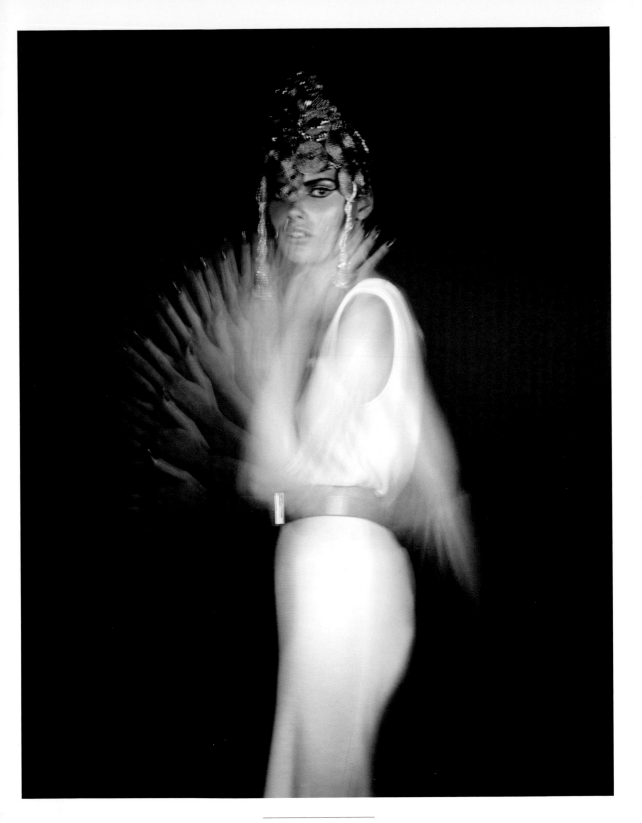

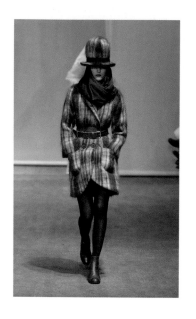

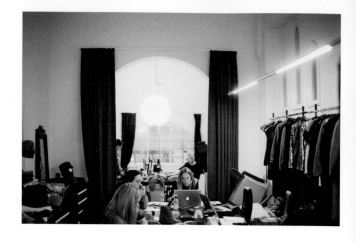

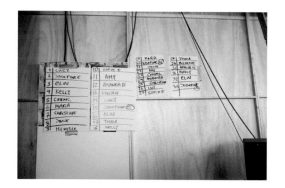

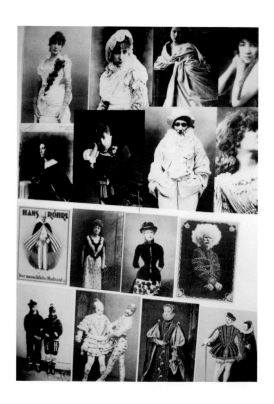

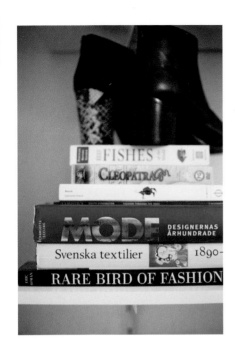

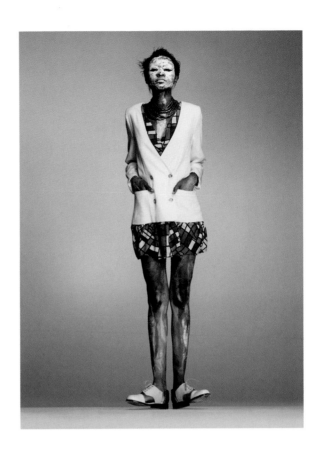

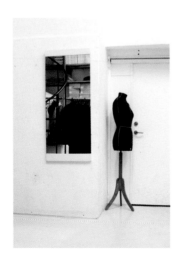

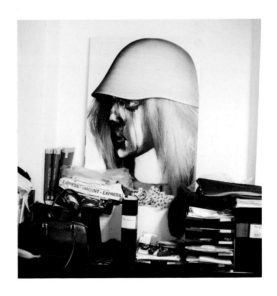

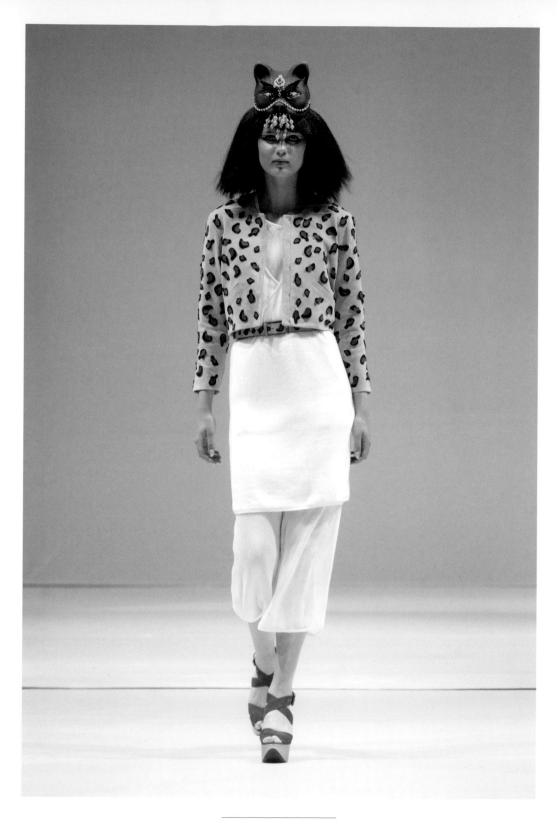

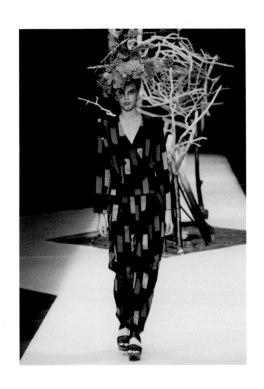

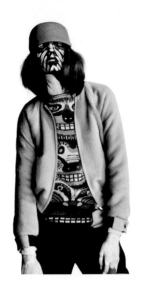

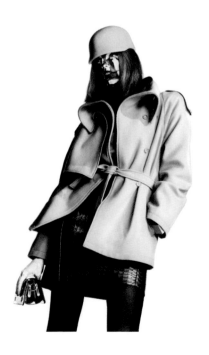

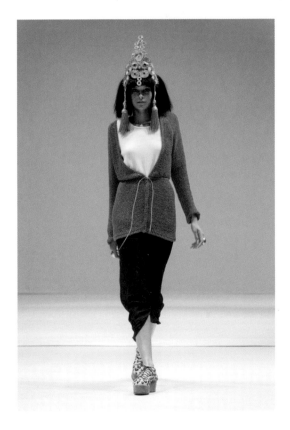

MOONSPOON SALOON

IT ALL STARTED WITH FOUR CREATIVES – ARTIST TAL R, DESIGNER SARA SACHS, PHOTOGRAPHER NOAM GRIEGST AND STYLIST MELANIE BUCHHAVE – WHO WANTED TO CREATE A BRAND WITH A NEW CONCEPT. TODAY THIS MOSTLY REVOLVES AROUND THE WORLD OF SARA SACHS, WHETHER THAT BE LOS ANGELES OR HER OWN HOMETOWN, COPENHAGEN. THE BRAND HAS NOTABLY PRESENTED ITSELF THROUGH PERFORMANCE WORK IN NEW YORK, COPENHAGEN AND LONDON.

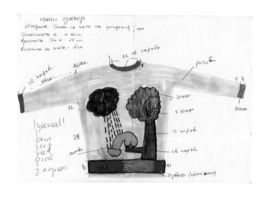

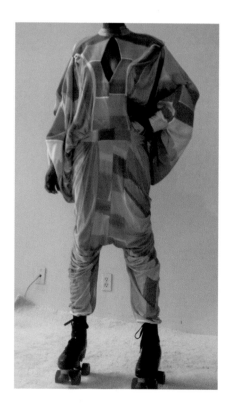

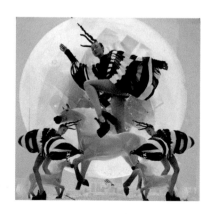

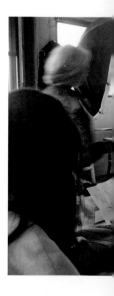

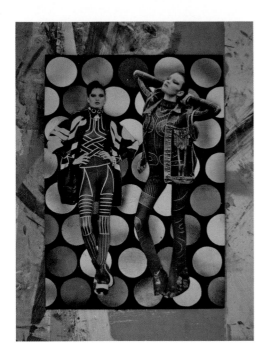

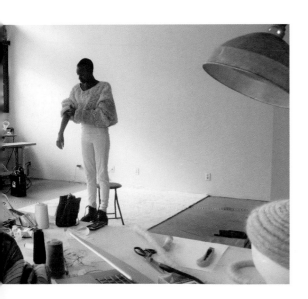

Sara, tell me about the concept of Moonspoon Saloon.
Moonspoon Saloon is fashion performance, combining powers of expression in one. It is manifested in characters presented in performances. The collections are the pieces from the stage and their imaginary friends and family.

Are you based in Los Angeles now? If so, how has being there inspired your work? Los Angeles is a place where I feel I can express myself freely. Clothing is somehow an armour from reality, and LA is engaged in this war on many levels. It's a city that embraces fantasy and creativity with a peculiar naive spirit. At the same time it's a place where social reality is in your face. It's industrial, poor, rich, ethnic, ugly, sad, touching and full of hope and despair. The transparency of Western culture inspires me. Los Angeles is a very emotional city.

You previously showcased your collections during Copenhagen Fashion Week, but now mostly do presentations. Why did you change your form of presenting, and do you think a presentation has a better impact than a show? Clothing is nothing without a body, and in that sense fashion only happens when somebody wears it. It's not like a painting you can hang on the wall. For me a show isn't a presentation of clothing; it's the moment of creation. Something is born and later it will walk the streets on strangers and live its own life. That is perhaps the real magic of fashion. We experimented with the form of presentation from the very first show at the Royal Theatre in Copenhagen, and it's grown into something that is more connected to performance art than to the catwalk. Since our performance at the Museum of Contemporary Art in Los Angeles, we have mostly worked with museums and galleries. We did a performance for the Armory Show in New York and we've also shown a piece at the gallery of Charlottenborg Palace in Copenhagen.

How do the four of you interact and communicate your ideas into the brand? Who does what? Moonspoon was founded by Tal R and Noam, but today I work with many different artists so it's not really a collective brand any longer. Melanie still styles the shows and Noam sometimes takes the pictures, and my work with Tal R is more about the creative and consistent, which is harder to do now since I live in Los Angeles.

How do you produce your pieces? Are they one-offs or made in a factory? Moonspoon Saloon started out with an odd concept of 99 pieces made in 99 unique editions. We had sweaters knitted by elderly women in old people's homes from

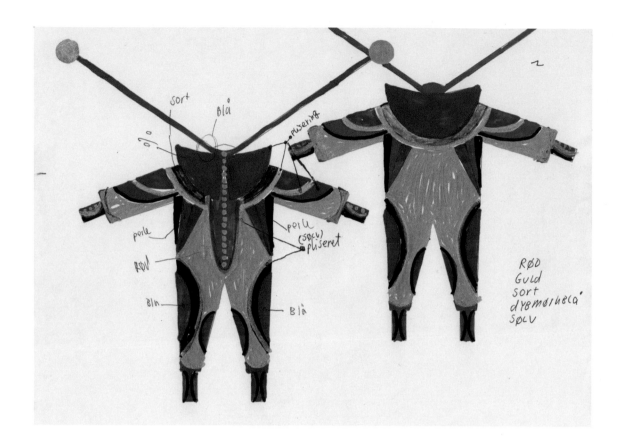

incorrect patterns and ancient tailors in the Czech mountains on the production line. It has changed a bit, but we still do most of our production in the Czech mountains and downtown Los Angeles. We've explored the ready-to-wear markets, but the heart of Moonspoon Saloon is couture. Our main focus now is unique pieces in fur, leather and silk, but we will continue to make products that are more accessible, like our shoe line.

How do you create those giant coloured furs? We worked with Saga Furs in the past, but we've just hired a furrier and will begin to produce our own in-house.

Where does your inspiration come from? I'm inspired by everything all the time. I was born like that, and the challenge for me is to navigate in this sea of inspiration.

What has been the most significant thing that has happened for the brand, and what are you planning for the future? For me the performance work stands out. It's the place where everything comes together. For a moment the armour is dropped and reality fades away. I want to do more and bigger performances, while making a stronger bond between the performances and the collections.

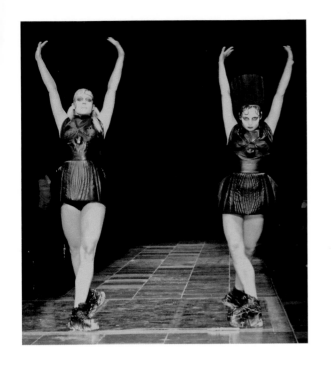

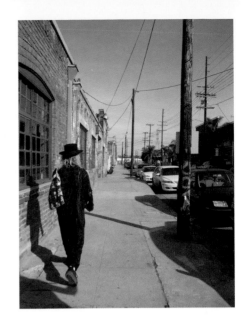

Opposite: Drawing by Tal R.

Above: Designer Sara Sachs in Los Angeles.

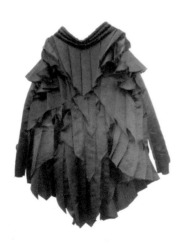

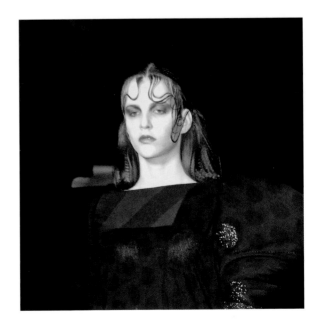

MUNDI

OUTLANDISH IDEAS, INSTALLATIONS AND KNITWEAR COULD SUM UP
MUNDI, BUT THIS ICELANDIC DESIGNER IS ALWAYS UNPREDICTABLE. WHETHER HE IS
DESIGNING THE ICELANDIC PHONE BOOK WITH THE USE OF KNITTED SPACEMEN OR BEING
BEATEN UP BY PEOPLE IN SUITS IN HIS ART INSTALLATIONS, THIS CREATIVE SPIRIT IS INVOLVED
IN MANY PROJECTS … NOT LEAST OF WHICH IS SELLING HIS FASHION COLLECTION
TO STORES AROUND THE WORLD DURING PARIS FASHION WEEK.

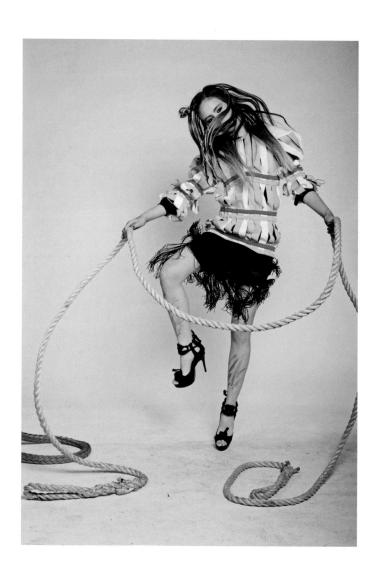

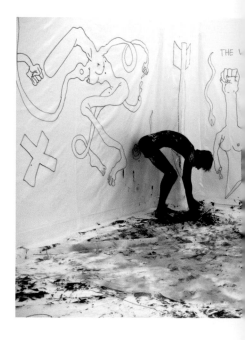

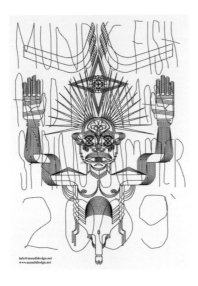

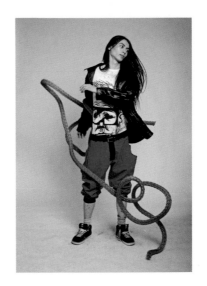

Above: Poster and artwork by Mundi.

Below: 'Chamber vs. Mundi' performance.

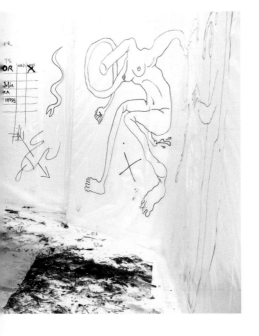

Tell me about the beginning of your brand. There was a contest at my art school to design the cover of the Icelandic phone book. I decided to use classic knit patterns, together with an image I'd been making in pixels of spacemen holding hands. When I went to the factory where they were making the knits and saw the spaceman fabric, I thought it would look great on a sweater. I drew on a piece of paper in the factory and later that same day it was ready! People started asking me where they could buy it so I asked KronKron, a concept store here in Reykjavik, if they would like to sell it. Before I knew it people started writing about it in newspapers and magazines, so after doing a few more versions I put together a collection and took it to Paris to show at 'Rendez-Vous', which is a collective show-room for new designers. My first season went straight into ten concept stores around the world – Tokyo, Berlin, Italy, New York, Paris – but I've been struggling in the fashion industry ever since!

How has being from Iceland influenced your designs? Well, Iceland being the place I've lived all my life has had a big impact on who I am. I believe you are much more influenced by your environment than you realize, so what you say and think are based on the environment around you. I'm not only talking about nature or houses. Experiences and discussions with people affect where your ideas come from. So we are never truly in control of ourselves. Please don't take your life too seriously because it's kind of a big joke and if you don't get it you won't have any fun…

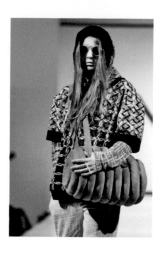

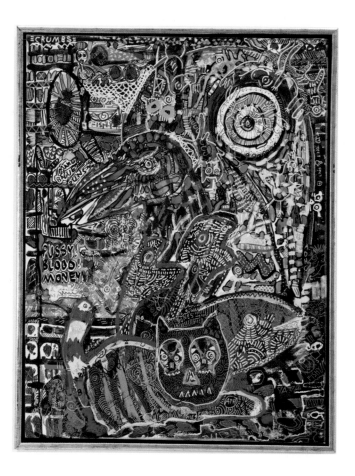

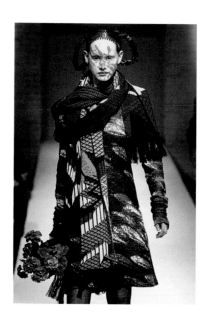

Left: Artwork by Mundi, Morri & Raggi ('Moms').

'I'm not into strong concepts anymore'

ON INSPIRATION

You seem to do a lot of installation art. How do you combine that with designing a collection? It is quite hard to combine fashion and art. Fashion will always need some sense of beauty. But there are a lot of mixed opinions, which is something I try to play with as much as possible. Variation is one of the fundamental elements of happiness. It's quite easy to stir fashion people because they're so used to a plain catwalk, which many of them dislike. To reach a good art opinion I must go much further. I think the best thing I've done is that I got six volunteers to fight me wearing my suits. The print turned out to be quite beautiful but the performance was quite rough and ugly.

I remember seeing a show of yours in Iceland where you used people on the catwalk who had a disorder. Some people were quite outraged by this, but as models they seemed to have such a good time and have so much character. Why did you choose to do this? I contacted the mothers of children who had Down's Syndrome. I've always liked people with this disorder because they're happy, carefree, strong and beautiful. Their personalities are rich and lively, and they have dreams and wishes to participate in life, society and the culture they live in and admire. When I asked the families if they wanted to be involved in my performance they were overwhelmed with happiness and excitement. They are so full of love that every chance they get they give you a hug and hug each other. Each one had a unique way of walking the catwalk — some danced and others clapped — but they all had one thing in common: they were super-happy. For those who think I was doing something wrong, they should look at the models on regular modern catwalks. Some of them almost seem to be falling apart with the pressure and confused ideas about what a normal person should look like.

What are you inspired by when you design? A lot of things, I guess. Mostly it comes out as I start working on the designs. I start by making the textiles, which are often an experiment with knitted graphics and messages. My first collections had very strong concepts, like 'The Guts of our Forefathers', which was inspired by blood, lungs, hearts and veins. I'm not into those strong concepts anymore and I like to keep it more abstract. I'm looking more at a feeling or an effect than a strong link to icons of something you might or might not know.

Tell me about your work process. I spend a lot of time just thinking and trying to visualize something effective before I start. After I design the fabrics, we have them produced and then we sew them together. When the fabrics arrive, it can be stressful to wrap up the collection, but making the textiles is really the most time-consuming part.

Is anything produced locally in Iceland? We have our own workshop, or sewing 'factory', where we try to do most of the work — at least all the prototypes. Then we outsource some items to Icelandic factories. We also use an Icelandic knitting factory as much as we can, but there is a lack of machines in Iceland. We have manufacturers for knitwear in Estonia and Turkey. They knit the fabrics that are not available in Iceland due to complex texture and yarn. We have to do complex cuts abroad as well.

Where do you see yourself in the future? Well, it's in the hands of commercial space engineers — whether or not they make it possible for me to get to space! But I'm a bit scared that might take longer than my lifetime, so I will have to wander the seven seas until then.

PETER JENSEN

DANISH SWEETHEART PETER JENSEN IS ONE OF SCANDINAVIA'S LEADING
CONTEMPORARY DESIGNERS. HIS GLOBAL STOCKISTS INCLUDE DOVER STREET MARKET
IN LONDON, SIDE BY SIDE IN TOKYO AND OPENING CEREMONY IN NEW YORK. HE HAS ALSO
DESIGNED CAPSULE COLLECTIONS FOR TOPSHOP/TOPMAN, FRED PERRY, WEEKDAY AND B STORE.
IN 2009 HE WAS THE RECIPIENT OF A £100,000 AWARD FROM THE DANISH ARTS COUNCIL,
AND IN 2010 HE WAS NOMINATED FOR THE SCOTTISH FASHION AWARDS. HE TEACHES
ON THE MA COURSE AT CENTRAL SAINT MARTINS IN HIS 'SPARE TIME'!

Tell me about the beginning of your brand. It was something that happened by mistake when I was finishing my MA at Central Saint Martins. Eo Bocci, an Italian company, came to the college and looked at ten of us, eight in womenswear and two in menswear. They were looking for a new designer – with money and a production deal. I thought, 'Well, I have no hope in hell, I'm menswear', and all the womenswear designers were always the ones more in focus. But they chose me, which was such a surprise. I was with them for three seasons, had a show in Paris, and then I left. I would have preferred to go out and work for someone, learn about the business and see what kind of mistakes you make when you have your own. But here we are, thirteen years down the line, happy as Larry…

The universe that you translate through your brand is so recognizable. Where does it come from? Well, I think directly from me. That is a short answer, but the truth.

Are you inspired by anything Scandinavian? I think that it's in my blood somehow, no? I can't really get away from where I come from, which is good, and I do think it has some kind of influence on how I view the world and the way I design. I'm happy to be from Scandinavia, but also very happy that I live in London. It's a very good combo.

You decided to be based in London. It is of course the hub of creativity, but why do you prefer that to having a studio in Denmark? Because it's too expensive to live in Denmark and do what I do, and I like the English way of working; it makes sense to me. There are so many rules in Denmark that can be hard to get around.

Do you feel more British than Scandinavian, having spent so many years abroad? I don't know if I feel one or the other. I can see good and bad in both cultures, and I think it's great that I can.

You also teach at Central Saint Martins. Did [head of MA fashion] Louise Wilson approach you about the opportunity? And how do you have the time?! Louise asked me if I wanted to come and look at the students' work. That was in 2001. I don't know how I have time to do it but it is something I enjoy, and I of course have a great team in the studio that I trust and that I know will be doing their work when I'm not there.

Do you get inspired by the students, or do you feel that you grow from being surrounded by a new generation? I've always said that the best feeling is if you get a student that you're jealous of. When one of the students presents you with a totally new concept, you go away knowing that you have done your job.

You have also published a book. Tell me about that project. We had our ten-year anniversary in 2011 and we knew that we wanted to do something special. We started talking and the idea of a book came along. It was great to go back over all the work we did in the first ten years, put it all together and get some of the people that we've worked with to be part of the book, like the graphic group Aabake, who we've been working with from the very beginning. We got Emily King and Susannah Frankel to write a piece. I'm very proud of and happy with it, and that we made it happen.

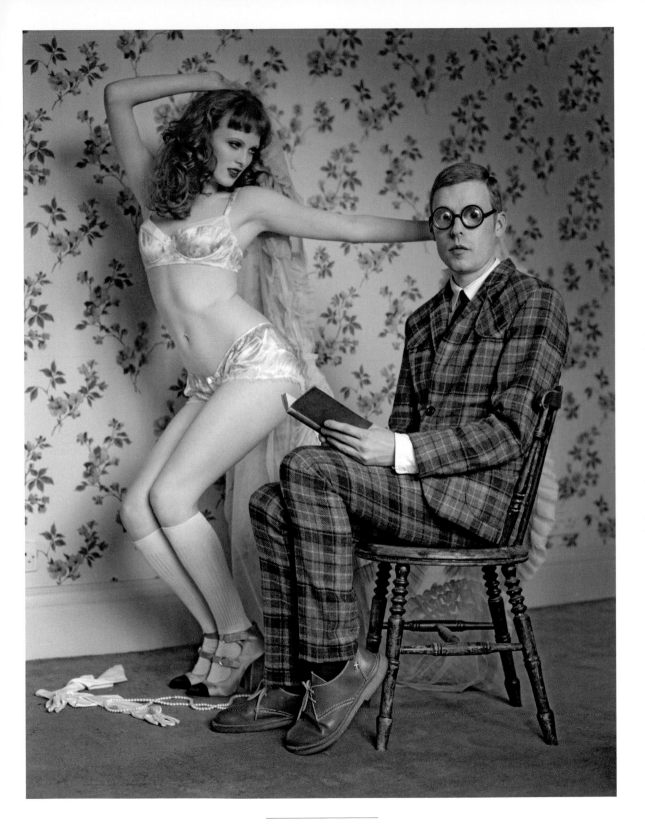

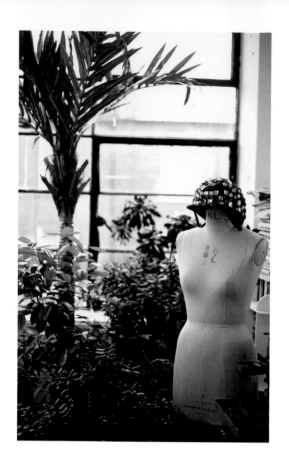

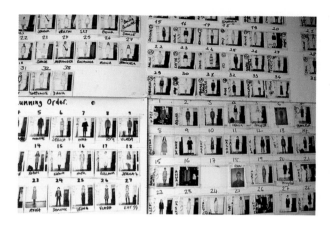

Left and below:
The atelier in east London.

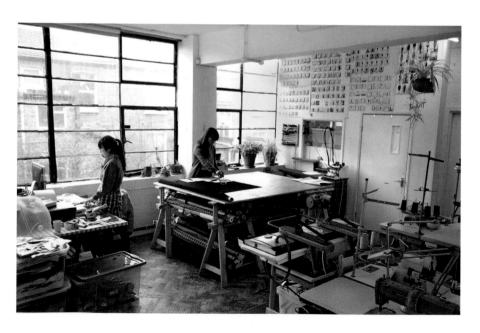

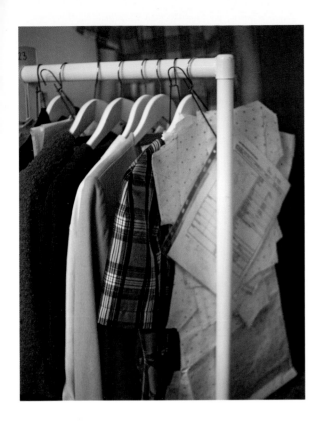

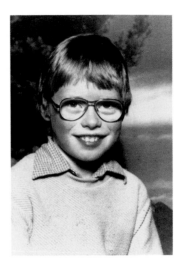

Above: Peter Jensen
as a child.

You seem to work from a muse. How do you find one each season, and who are some of your favourite ones of the past? I like women, but I also think that they are way more complicated than men, and I think that is something that I like in all the so-called muses/women that we've used in the collections. It makes it easy for me to talk to my team about what my thoughts are with each collection. I see them as a working tool. I don't think I have a favourite, but some of them have been easier to work around/with than others.

Please tell me about the rabbit because it appears in a lot of your designs. There's not that much to tell about the rabbit! It was a graphic print that we used in the second

collection – SS02 'Mildred'. It was, and is, just a perfect little thing to use as a brand logo and to play around with in other elements, like on a T-shirt, a bag, etc.

Where is your collection manufactured? Do you source anything locally? We get 60% produced in the UK, because I like the fact that we can support the industry in the country where we are based. There's something great about the fact that it has a label saying 'Made in England'. I like that.

What will happen in the future for Peter Jensen? Are you staying in London? Yes, I have no plans to move anywhere. I like living in the UK and I'm married to an Englishman.

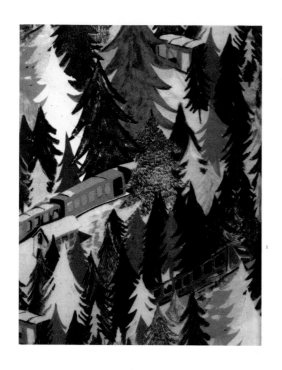

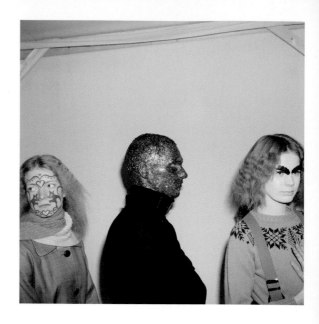

Left: Collage work for a print.

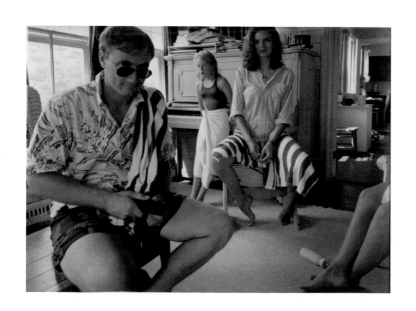

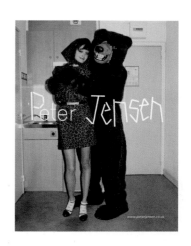

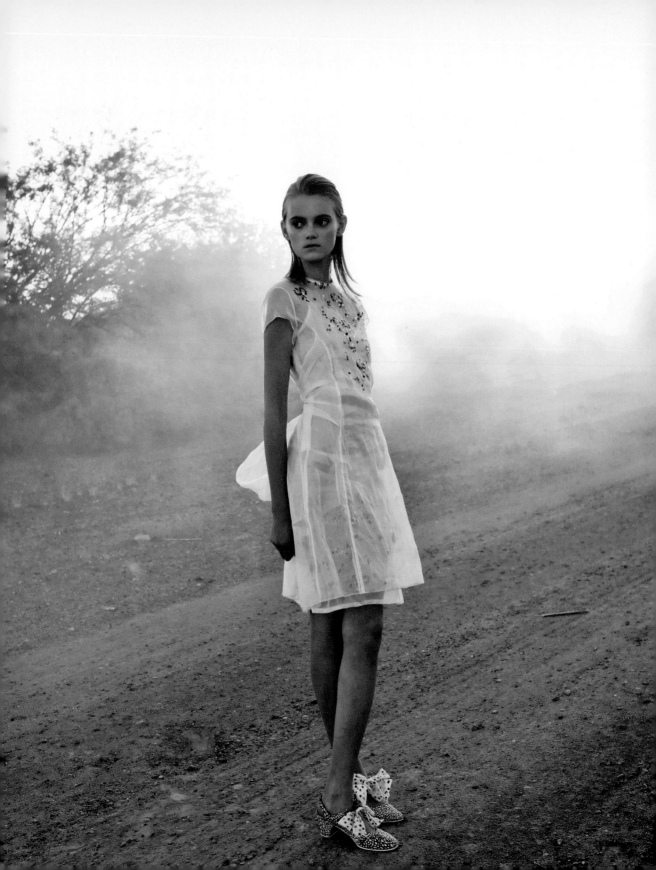

R/H

TWO FRIENDS FROM FINLAND – HANNA RIIHELÄINEN AND EMILIA HERNESNIEMI –
STARTED THEIR BRAND IN 2010 AFTER WORKING AT ZAC POSEN AND AGENCY V AND
AFTER 6 YEARS OF STUDYING. RISK-TAKERS FROM THE MTV GENERATION, THEY ARE INSPIRED
BY LIFE AROUND THEM – FROM DRAGONS TO FEMALE ANATOMY. THEIR DESIGNS
CAN BE FOUND IN MORE THAN 25 RETAILERS AROUND THE WORLD
AND IN THEIR OWN BOUTIQUE, R/H MINI SHOP, IN HELSINKI.

Tell me about the name of your brand. Where does it come from? The name of the label – R/H – comes from our last names. We met while studying at the University of Art & Design Helsinki, and our first name as a duo was Riiheläinen-Hernesniemi. Too bad Finnish names are just a bit too tricky for the international market! We decided to make it a bit simpler. We like the name for its kind of masculine simplicity.

What was it like growing up in Finland? We both grew up in very different parts of the country. Although Finland`s population is only a bit over five million, geographically it is a large country and the north is far from the south. Emilia grew up in the north in a little city called Oulu, far away from fashion or anything really cool. Hanna grew up on an island called Laajasalo to the east of Helsinki. We both experienced typical suburban childhoods, with big yards, lots of forest, lots of friends and pranks. We were both born in the 1980s and Finland looked quite different back then. We both share the feeling of being on the edge of the world and finding exotic things via MTV, music, magazines and American TV series, such as *Knight Rider*, *Baywatch*, *Dallas*, *Beverly Hills 90210* and *Dynasty*.

When did you decide to launch the label together? We studied a long time together – six years! We finished school with MAs in 2009. We got to know each other better quite late, maybe in the third or fourth year. Coming from Finland it was obvious to us that there weren't really jobs we could apply for after leaving school. Also we both have a thing for taking risks and seeing how far we can go. So the theme of our Masters thesis was Riiheläinen-Hernesniemi as a collection and a brand. We wrote down what we wanted to achieve and how we were going to do it. It still serves as a basis for the label, but of course

we had no idea how much work it really is developing a base for a sustainable company and a visual line. After graduation we worked for a bit. Then we launched R/H in July 2010, with our first season being SS11.

Do you work in a large team or by yourselves? We work with two wonderful Russian professionals here in Helsinki – Irja as our pattern maker, Janina as our dressmaker. We make all of our samples in Finland and in Estonia. In the company there are only the two of us, Hanna and Emilia, but we use a lot of outside help, buying most of the services, so that explains the small number of employees.

Hanna, you worked at Zac Posen in New York and, Emilia, you worked in PR at Agency V in Berlin. That must be quite a perfect combination of creative know-how and press knowledge. Where are you based now, and what does a normal day look like for you? We are based in Helsinki, but of course we dream of changing scene again some day. Our normal days seem to be crazy in a good way at the moment. Then again we don't know any entrepreneur labels whose days would be 9 to 5. As we are the only employed people, we stretch our limits all the time, doing everything from design to selling, packing and delivering. We already have about 25 retailers around Europe and the US, and we can only thank ourselves for that. Right now we are spending a lot of time doing interviews and replying to emails. It is hard to find a moment with us both designing something. Our most normal day is a day at the computer or in our shop, contacting old and new customers, finding fabrics and searching for our printed fabrics, which always seem to get lost on their way from Germany to Finland!

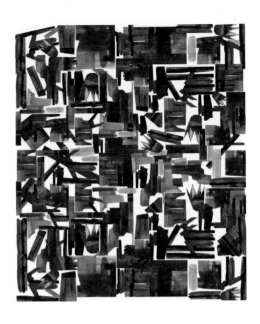

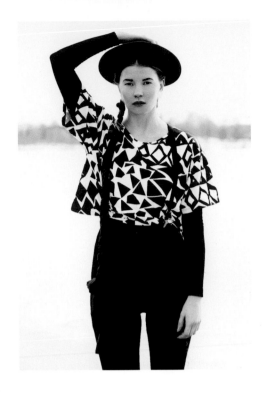

Above: Stripes multicolour print from the AW11 collection.

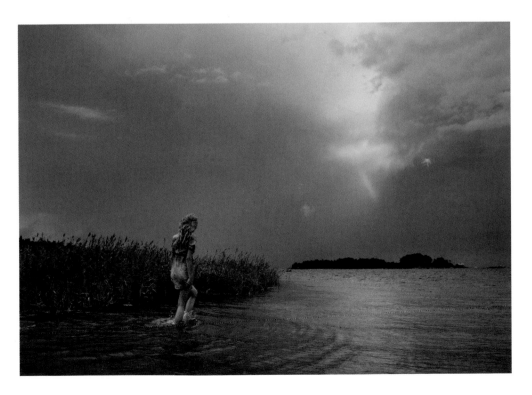

'Inspiration can start from a picture that you see while walking somewhere, or a granny's hat that you see on the tram'

ON INSPIRATION

You haven't been around for that long but you already have quite a few shops representing your brand. Tell me a bit about where we can find your designs. We will be at International Playground in New York and Wald in Berlin. We hope to keep our spot at Henrik Vibskov Boutique and U.S. Import in Copenhagen. We also hope to find a perfect shop in Sweden (it seems a bit hard coming from Finland). In Finland you will definitely find us at the R/H MINI SHOP in the centre of Helsinki, and hopefully also at the department store Stockmann, where R/H now has a full mini-department. Even in the smaller cities in Finland we have some really nice shops, like Busstop in Rauma and Pohjan Some in Oulu. There are beautiful webshops that sell R/H as well, like our own shop, rh-the-label.com, but also a fresh new webshop called acolyth. com, and finnishdesignshop.com.

What are you inspired by in your collections? Inspiration can come from mixtures of very different things and moods. It can start from a picture that you see while walking somewhere, or a granny's hat that you see on the tram. You need to experience different periods or decades, listen to old and new music, be open to different underground cultures, and just search for things that can shake your world. One good picture or feeling can be the key for the collection if it's the one for you. Our inspiration comes from the world and atmosphere that we live in. It can come from contrasts, such as nature/city, rough/playful and black/colourful. Anatomy is also something that has been very important for all the R/H collections. To get the best cuts for different pieces you must be inspired by the female anatomy. R/H's collections have also been inspired by the cosmos, astronauts, dragons, mountains, Mickey Mouse, eyes, Russian ladies working in fields, space and a female knight, just to mention a few things!

Do you get your garments produced in Finland? R/H produces some samples and all of its jewelry in Helsinki, but almost everything else is produced in Tallinn, Estonia, at the moment. The factory is the closest that we have to our studio in Helsinki. It is only around 80 km away. It's nice to know the people who sew our pieces, and we have a very good relationship with the factory.

What are your goals for the future? Our goal is to develop R/H in the right direction, making good decisions and taking care of each other. R/H should also keep its own look, colours, prints, quality and silhouettes. We want to be inspired by life happening around us and to us. We hope to find a healthy sustainability concerning the label and its balance.

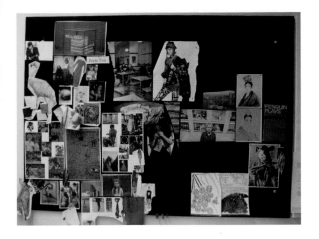

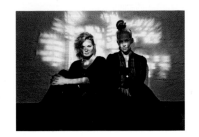

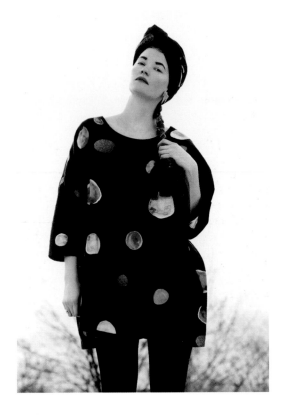

Above right: designers Hanna
Riiheläinen and Emilia Hernesniemi.

Below right: R/H Mini Shop
in Helsinki.

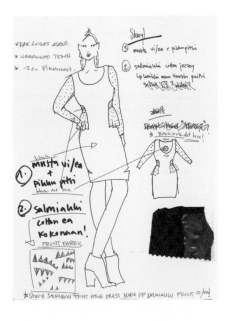

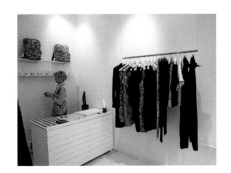

RIIS

THE DANISH DESIGNER STINE RIIS IS VERY BUSY. SHE HAD ONLY RECENTLY GRADUATED FROM LONDON COLLEGE OF FASHION WHEN SHE WON THE INTERNATIONAL H&M DESIGN AWARD, WHICH ATTRACTED CONTESTANTS FROM 14 OF THE MOST PRESTIGIOUS DESIGN SCHOOLS IN SWEDEN, THE UK, GERMANY, BELGIUM, HOLLAND AND DENMARK. HER FUTURE LOOKS BRIGHT.

Tell me about the beginning of your brand. My brand is very much newborn and still developing. I graduated in June 2011 and my graduation collection – AW12 'Decadence & Decay' – was my first collection.

What did you study? I studied Fashion Design Technology Womenswear at London College of Fashion.

Whereabouts in Denmark did you grow up, and did you feel inspired by the country at all for your collection? I grew up in the south of Jutland, just half an hour from the German border, in a small town of 4,000 inhabitants. I can't ignore the legacy of Danish design; it's a part of who I am, which reflects my aesthetics. I get inspired by Danish modern furniture. I like simplicity with subtle details, and I like to mix different colours and textures. I tend to invest in garments that I know I will love to wear for years – just as you can look at a couch by the designer Finn Juhl and never get tired of it.

Where do you manufacture your garments? At the moment I'm sourcing manufacturers in Europe for my next collection. Up until now I've made everything myself as I couldn't afford a tailor and wanted to get as good at sewing as possible.

Do you get anything produced locally? No, unfortunately not. I would love to do some locally produced knits in the future, but at the moment my company is too small for that option.

How do you think young designers finance a brand like your own? They work hard!

What has been the highlight of your career thus far? Winning the H&M Design Award 2012. It's been a great experience, and I couldn't imagine a better start to my career as a designer. The €50,000 has given me the opportunity to work towards my own vision as a designer. Hilary Alexander [at *The Daily Telegraph*], Christopher Kane and Kristopher Arden-Houser [at *Vogue* Italia] were judges in the competition and, by choosing me as the winner, showed that they believed in my vision, which has given me the recognition and motivation to start my own label. A part of the experience in connection with the H&M Award was my own huge fashion show at Stockholm Fashion Week. Iris Strubegger walked my show – a dream come true, as she was an inspiration for the collection.

Tell me about your working process. Where do you start when you need inspiration, and what happens then? My radar for inspiration is constantly turned on. I'm a very curious person and I like to explore anything new. I try to stay up to date on contemporary art, photography, architecture, lifestyle, food, politics and general trends in society. My initial ideas usually come from a mix of inputs from different channels and take form almost subconsciously. When I've defined a direction, I start to drape on the stand and toile the initial shapes. At the same time I sketch and do fabric experiments. From then on I develop details, such as a cuff, a collar, a button-stand or pocket, and perfect the shapes.

You are still at an early stage in your career, but do you have anything planned for the future? At the moment I'm really excited to be working on my first spring collection. Then at the beginning of fall my collection 'Decadence & Decay' will be sold in selected H&M stores in Denmark, Germany, Belgium, England, Sweden and the Netherlands. I'm very much looking forward to seeing my designs on the street.

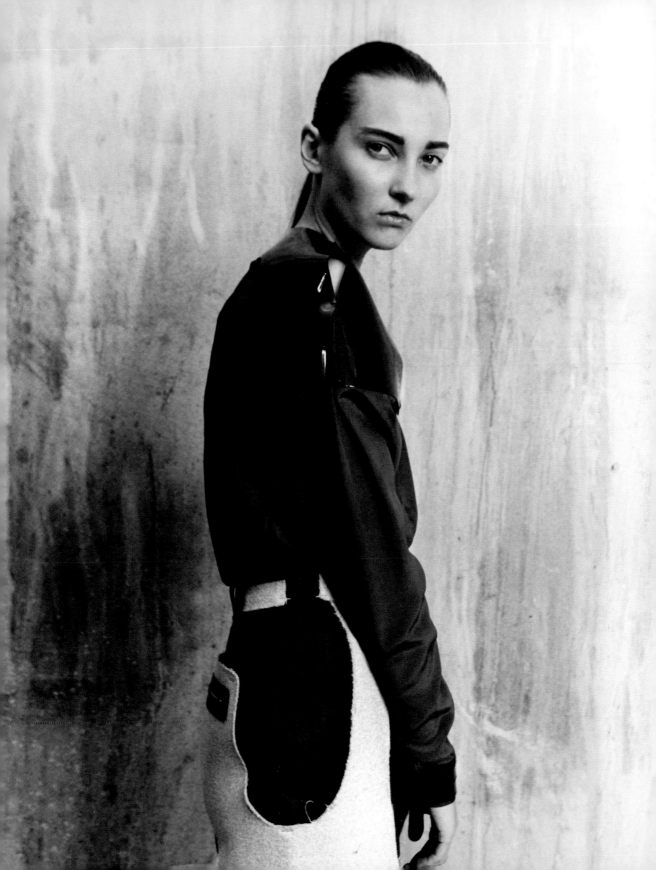

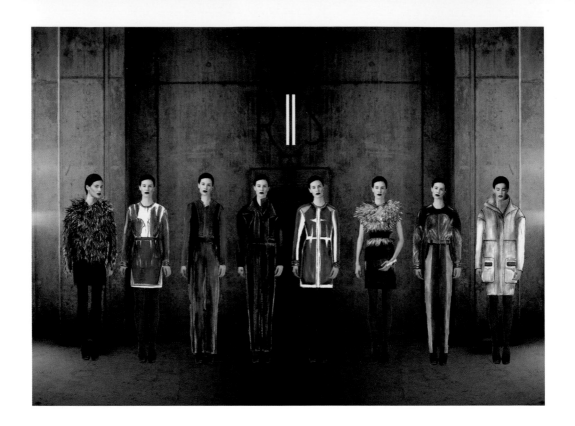

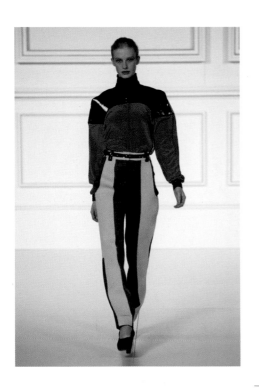

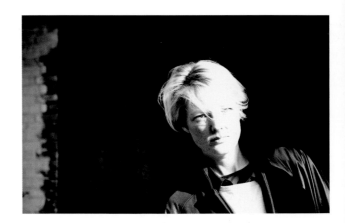

Above: Designer Stine Riis.

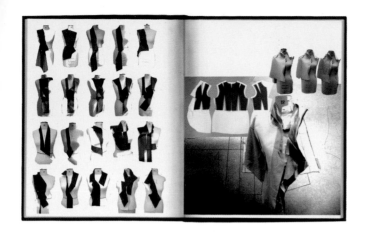

'My radar for inspiration is
constantly turned on. I'm a
very curious person and I like
to explore anything new'

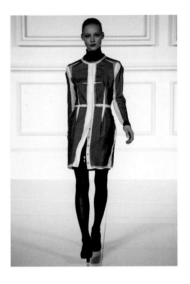

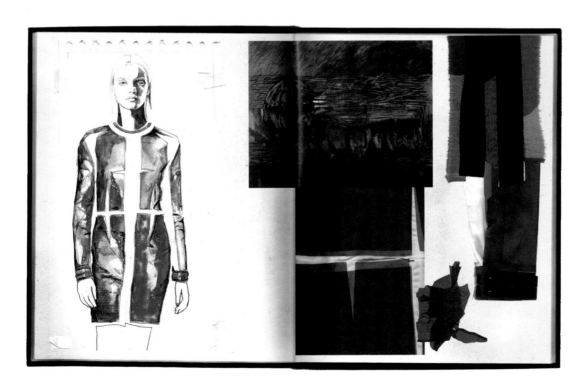

RÜTZOU

THERE IS SOMETHING OF THE FAIRYTALE ABOUT SUSANNE RÜTZOU. SHE GREW UP
WITH A NOMADIC MOTHER, SO SPENT A LOT OF TIME IN HER GRANDMOTHER'S ATELIER,
HIDING UNDER A DESK. TODAY HER BRAND IS ONE OF THE MOST RECOGNIZED DANISH LABELS,
WITH INTERNATIONAL SUCCESS AND FANS INCLUDING MODEL AND VOGUE BLOGGER
LAURA BAILEY. AS A WINNER OF THE SUSTAINABILITY DESIGN CHALLENGE AT THE
COPENHAGEN FASHION SUMMIT, SHE IS COMMITTED TO POSITIVE CHANGE.

Tell me about your upbringing and what led you into design. I was an only child and my parents got divorced when I was three or four years old. I lived with my mother, who was still very young and loved to travel all over the world for long periods of time. I therefore spent a lot of time with my grandparents, whom I adored, and I remember many long and lovely holidays in their summerhouse, being totally absorbed by drawing whole universes of imaginary characters. I would draw not just a girl in a pretty dress, but her whole wardrobe, her trunk and her airship, all carefully coordinated. When my mother presented me with a box of those drawings it was remarkable to see the red thread that has led to my work today.

Tell me about your grandmother. My grandmother was a couturier with her own studio and a small but exclusive clientele. It was at the end of an era when women with resources would rather have their clothes made especially for them than buy them ready-made. I could spend whole days in her studio and I loved to hide under her big table, playing with her boxes of buttons and beautiful trimmings while watching the fittings. I was, however, always more interested in the process and the materials than in the big glamorous bridal gowns or evening dresses, which were hung up among the chandeliers. I was a child with a strong will and from an early age had specific ideas about what I would wear. My mother soon got tired of our discussions and gave me a budget. It didn't go very well and my grandmother was always my salvation when winter came and I had spent all the money. She would let me design a coat by myself and we would choose the fabric together, and I would assist her and watch her make it. It is probably more than anything those moments with her that later made it such a natural choice for me to channel my creativity into fashion and design.

You also seem to take a bit of inspiration from the art world. Do you travel a lot outside of Scandinavia when you need inspiration? Yes, art is an important source of inspiration. The abstract energy triggers my creativity and transforms it into new images within my personal universe. I use it for textural effects and for sentiments in a collection. There is also an inexhaustible source of colour inspiration to be found in the art world. I tend to spend a lot of time on exhibitions, especially when in Paris, London or New York. Other favourite destinations include Tokyo, and various parts of India and Africa. I, however, no longer feel the urge to implement the ethnic element in my work, and the inspiration I get from travelling is mostly indirect.

Do you start by drawing? How does everything come together? It always starts with time for reflection and research. I try to define my intuitive approach for a new season. I write a lot down and hang up images everywhere in our studio. After a while we edit it all into a more precise mood board and continue with colours, prints, fabrics and loose sketches. Only then, when almost everything is settled, will I start to draw and specify the details.

Model and *Vogue* contributor Laura Bailey fell in love with your clothes. What do you think makes your brand so successful? Bless her! I think it's because my clothes relate to the lives many urban women live today. The design is seemingly simple but feminine, often with quirky details, which allow the wearer's own personality to shine through and enable them to combine the garments in various ways and to keep them relevant in their wardrobe for a long time. We also deliberately keep our collections at relatively accessible prices.

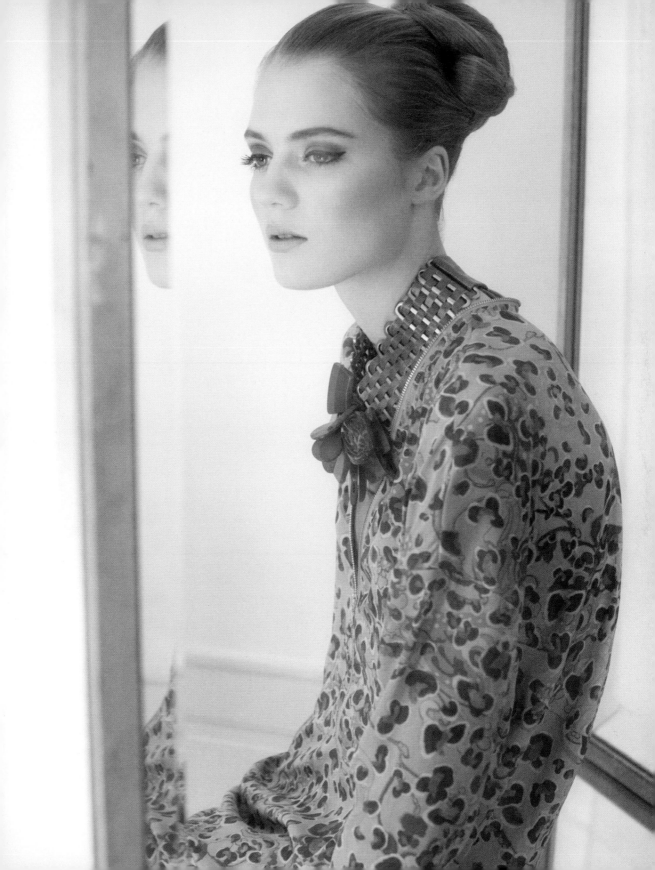

'Art is an important source of inspiration. The abstract energy triggers my creativity and transforms it into new images within my personal universe'

ON INSPIRATION

You were invited to participate in a design challenge during the Copenhagen Fashion Summit 2012, using only sustainable textiles … and you won. Tell me about the process with those designs. It is wonderfully refreshing sometimes to work on a project that doesn't relate to the normal collection cycle. My team and I enjoyed ourselves tremendously, getting our hands into tea dyes, draping on mannequins and working freely and intuitively within a sustainable frame. The inspiration was mainly taken from a selection of images from Edward Burtynsky's amazingly beautiful book, *Oil*. I was determined to end up with an expression that not only showed the essence of Rützou's design DNA but also emphasized the fact that sustainable fashion can still be poetic and sensual. Obviously, we were very pleased that we also ended up winning the challenge, but moreover I was very happy that the summit itself turned out to be a great success. It was a highly inspiring and enlightening day, with speakers from all over the world focusing on the fact that the fashion world has to take its responsibilities seriously, and the sooner the better.

Has the experience made you want to use more sustainable fabrics and resources? The way I see it, there's no choice. The fashion industry is the fourth most polluting industry in the world, so in order to save the planet and make sure our children have a healthy environment to grow up in, we have to change. The highly frustrating part is that, even though we would like to implement a much higher degree of sustainability in our collections, it's not yet entirely accessible for companies our size. Good intentions, however, also make a difference, and sustainability is beginning to have an impact on the choices we make here at Rützou.

Your designs are also sold abroad. Do you think women outside of Scandinavia want to own a part of the Nordic style more today than before? And what has made it so popular, do you think? Increasing globalization is probably a part of the answer. Women all over the world tend more and more to relate to similar values, and so the way we express ourselves becomes more uniform. The Nordic approach to design, which generally seems to be relatively pragmatic and down to earth without compromising the aspect of articulation, is also very compatible with the ongoing recession. Accessibility and longevity are strong arguments everywhere these days.

What will happen to Rützou next? Being a medium-sized Danish brand, we still have a lot of work to do in order to be more firmly established and noticed throughout Europe. I am a strong believer in being focused and 'having our soul with us' in what we do, rather than spreading our energy in too many directions at the same time. On a more personal level, I'm looking forward to releasing the next issue of *The Rützou Chronicle*, and I'm also looking forward to finding out what impact airy new surroundings will have on my creative mind, as Rützou is about to move headquarters to a new space in the centre of Copenhagen.

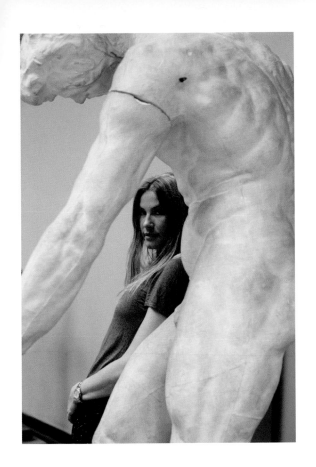

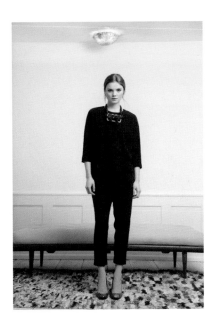

Left: Designer Susanne Rützou in the NY Carlsberg Glyptotek museum, Copenhagen.

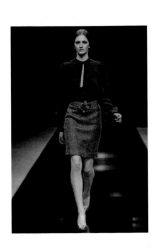

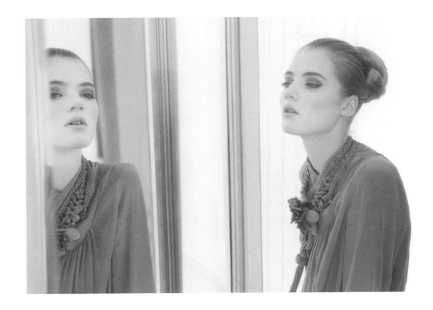

SAMUJI

THE SAMUJI BRAND WAS ESTABLISHED BY SAMU-JUSSI KOSKI, THE FORMER CREATIVE
DIRECTOR OF MARIMEKKO, BUT THERE IS NOW A SMALL TEAM, COMPLETE WITH DESIGNER
HENNAMARI ASUNTA, WORKING OUT OF HELSINKI. SUSTAINABILITY IS VERY IMPORTANT TO THE
COMPANY: ALL THE PRODUCTION UNITS AND MOST OF THE MATERIALS ARE FROM EUROPE.
THIS RELATIVE NEWCOMER, WITH AN INSPIRING WEBSITE, IS ONE TO WATCH.

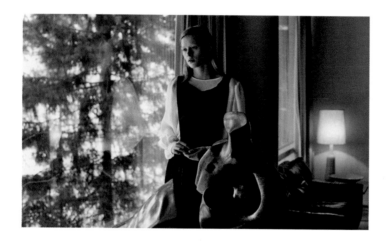

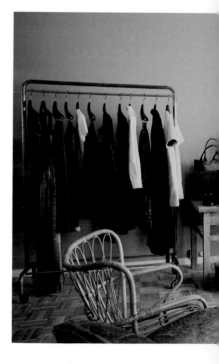

Below: The Samuji
showroom in Helsinki.

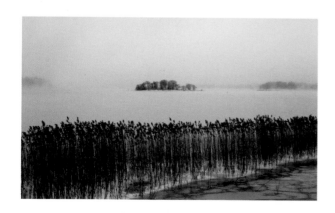

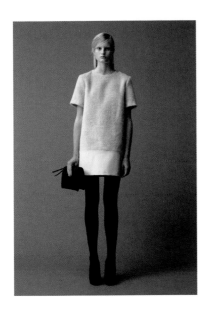

Suvi-Elina [Enqvist], in your role as stylist, can you tell me about the beginning of Samuji. It was established by Samu-Jussi Koski, who previously worked as the creative director of Marimekko, but wanted to start something of his own. Samuji was born out of the idea of having a place and medium for any type of creative project. It is thus a creative studio, but our main project at the moment is definitely our clothing line.

You are based in the old Vallila district of Helsinki. Tell me about the area. Vallila is an old residential area. The houses are small, cute and colourful, in pastel shades. There is also an area of wooden houses that is considered a national heritage.

How many of you are there in the company as a whole, and what is your daily routine? At the moment there are eleven of us. Since we're quite small, we're only in the early stages of having a strong routine. Basically we all do everything, even though we also have separate responsibilities or emphasis on certain aspects.

Why have you decided to design two separate lines? The two-line collection is based on women having so-called staple items, such as white shirts, tees, jeans, basic knitwear, etc. The idea is to colour the classic line with the styles of the seasonal collection.

You have selected manufacturers and suppliers. Are they based around where you live, or are they abroad? One of the Samuji values is to work as sustainably as possible. All our producers are in Europe — in Italy and Estonia. All our materials are also from Europe, with the exception of a couple of Japanese suppliers.

I love the video *Two Fifty Three* — beautiful music and landscape but very different, one being exotic and sensual, the other cold and distant. Is this how Finland feels and looks for you? It's quite tricky to reflect on how we as Finns perceive Finnishness. But — for sure — silence, wide open spaces, nature, cold and darkness are part of us. But at the same time we feel as if we have this very rich and colourful heritage, too, including the vibes from over the eastern border and old Karelia.

You are quite a new brand. What are you working on at the moment? We've started to work on our next collection. We also have quite a few collaborations and projects going on, keeping us very busy. More info on that soon…

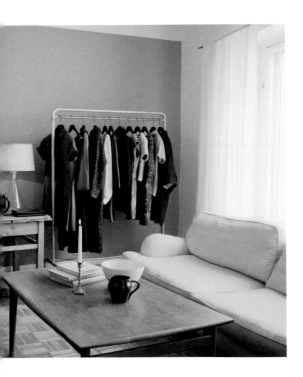

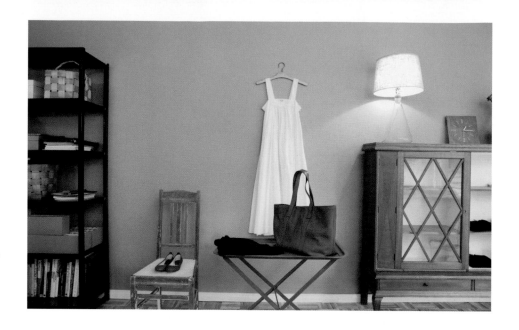

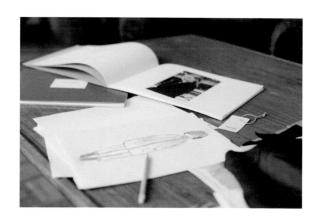

This page: Creative workspace
in the Vallila district of Helsinki.

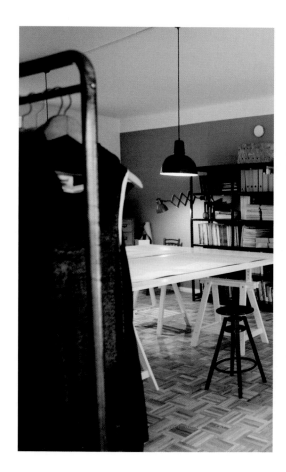

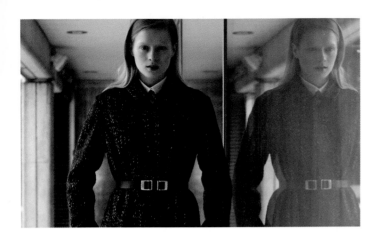

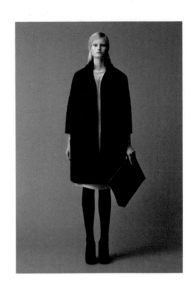

This page: Images from the Samuji campaign and lookbook, which have been released as a book.

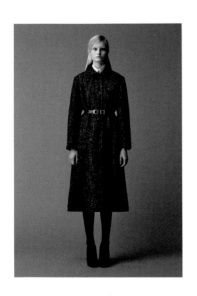

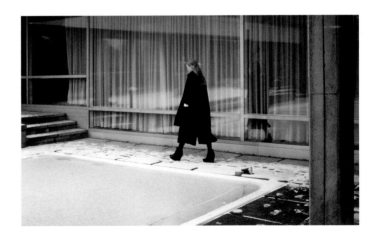

SANDRA BACKLUND

THIS ENIGMATIC DESIGNER LIVES AND WORKS JUST OUTSIDE OF STOCKHOLM. SHE HAS NO TEAM AND NO INTERNS, BUT, WITH THE HELP OF HER FAMILY, SHE DEDICATES HER TIME TO HER COMPANY, AND HAS MANAGED TO PRODUCE SOME OF THE MOST STUNNING GARMENTS, INCLUDING KNITWEAR, THAT SCANDINAVIA HAS TO OFFER.

Your garments are amazing. Do you produce everything in your studio? Most of the pieces I produce are handmade by me in my studio, but I've also done some test collaborations with a couple of Italian knitwear factories.

Do you use specialized machines for your knitwear, or are those pieces produced abroad? I work with a three-dimensional collage method, whereby I develop some basic hand-knitted bricks which I multiply and attach in different ways until they become a garment. When I collaborated with the production companies, we applied the same method but using basic knitting machines instead of hand-knitting.

Tell me about your upbringing. I grew up in quite a small, safe city in the north of Sweden and had a typical late 1970s/early 1980s Swedish childhood, with a lot of creative or sporty activities, often outdoors. I come from a simple and loving family. I was taught to be proud of who I am and where I come from, but I was encouraged to reach for more if I wanted it.

Did you grow up knowing that you wanted to do what you do now, or was it a slow process of evolution? I've always felt a strong connection towards arts and crafts and a need to express myself in a creative way, but I've also always had a strong theoretical and mathematical side. My whole life I've had hard times trying to make these two opposites cooperate, and I think I often took the easy way out, choosing only one of them while denying the other. Through the kind of fashion I do, I've finally found a way to combine both my free and my computing sides.

Do you feel that it is a struggle to be a designer and run a company? How do you manage? It is very difficult to be an independent designer, running your own company, but I try not to think too much about that. In the end I do this because I love the challenge, but of course it would be nice one day to be able to live off all the hard work.

It must be very time-consuming if you have to hand-knit some pieces. How do you have time to balance that and all the more boring business sides of running a company? To aim for balance right now is 'mission impossible'. I always feel as if I don't have enough time, especially for the creative process, but I do work all the time so somehow I still manage to handle the most crucial things.

You studied at Beckmans College of Design. Would you recommend this instead of people heading to London or New York for a design education? It's very difficult for me to say because I don't know the London or New York schools, but in general I always recommend Beckmans if someone asks for my opinion.

Did you intern anywhere? Your design is quite dramatic and not 'Scandinavian Minimal'. I'm wondering if you had a stint at Alexander McQueen or anything like that? No, I never interned anywhere. I graduated from fashion school in May 2004 and founded my own company and label the very same day.

Do you work with a big team or interns? Tell me about a normal day for you. I don't have a team and I never take on interns. Except for a long-term collaboration with my press office, Ibeyostudio, it's only me and my family running the business. A normal day for me is a 16-hour mish-mash of handicraft work, phone calls and emailing.

What kind of clients do you have for your couture pieces? A secret Daphne Guinness maybe? And where do you sell? Since I'm based a bit offside here in Stockholm

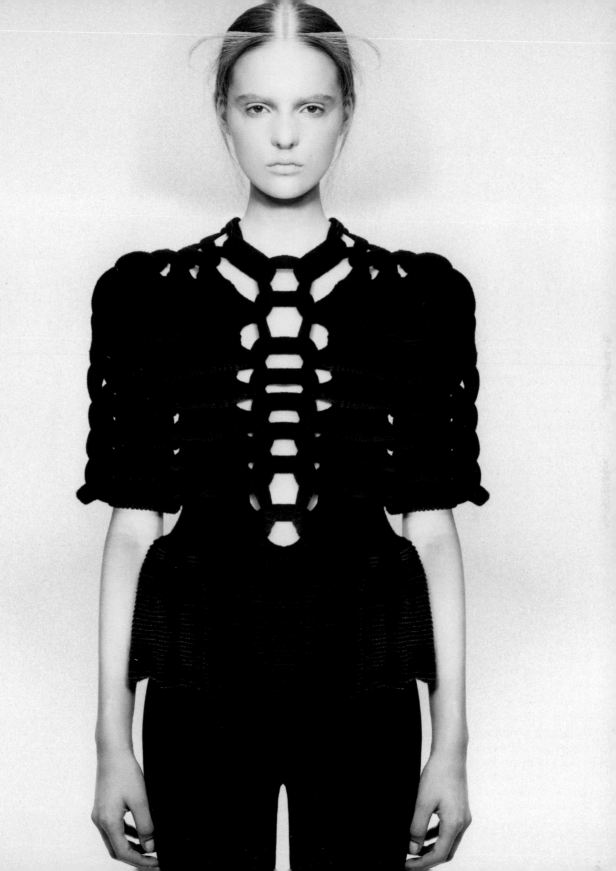

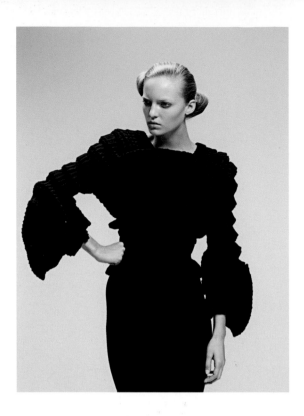

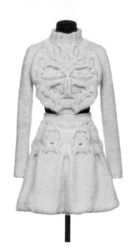

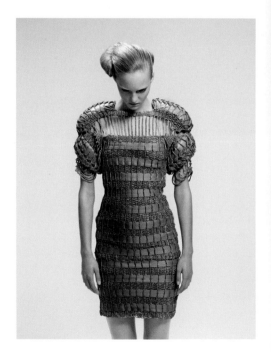

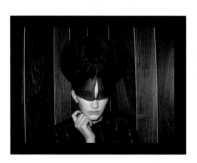

I never really meet my clients. Usually they contact me through my website and we discuss the order over email or phone, and then I custom-make the garments the old-fashioned way, made-to-measure. Apart from the private orders, I'm currently collaborating with the Antwerp store, Sien.

What are you working towards at the moment and over the next five years? I try to keep an open mind and not worry too much about the future. My only plan is to continue to work hard, protect my origins and what I'm good at, but still find a way to develop my designs and my company.

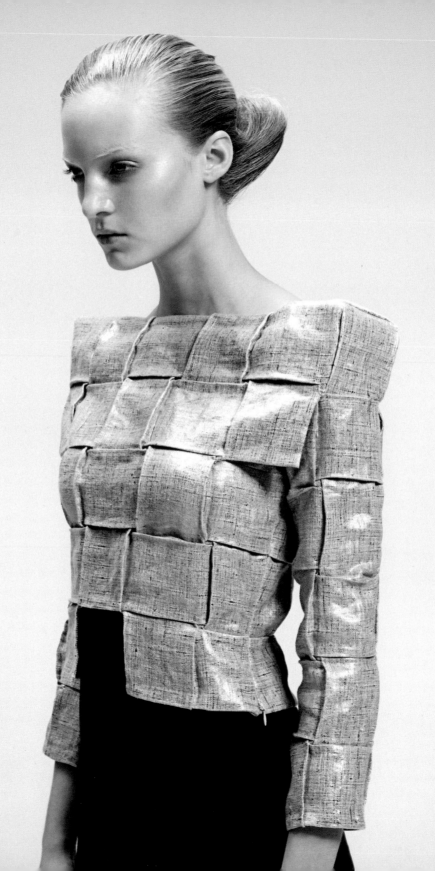

SOULLAND

SILAS ADLER'S INSPIRATION COMES FROM AMERICAN STREETWEAR, WHICH HE TURNS INTO URBAN FASHION-ORIENTED MENSWEAR. HE STARTED OUT DESIGNING A T-SHIRT LINE IN HIS KITCHEN, WITH HELP FROM HIS MOTHER, AND TODAY HIS COLLECTIONS ARE SOLD IN SOME OF THE MOST PRESTIGIOUS STORES IN THE WORLD. HE ALSO OWNS HIS OWN SHOP IN COPENHAGEN WITH A DESIGN STUDIO IN THE BACK.

Tell me about your upbringing. You're from Jutland, but later moved to Copenhagen? Well, it's a bit more complex than that. My mother is from Sweden and my father was from Tanzania. I was born in Aarhus in Jutland, but later moved to the countryside. When I was eight, my mother and I moved to Gothenburg in Sweden. We lived there until I was 12, and then we moved to Copenhagen. So despite having spent a good portion of my life elsewhere, I see Copenhagen as my hometown and as the city that raised me. I guess the place you are during your teenage years really becomes your base for the rest of your life – at least that's true for me.

When did you decide you wanted to launch a label? I think you were still young. That must have been challenging. I started when I was 17, from one day to the next. I didn't know anything and had no experience, so in that sense the beginning wasn't that hard, but then along the way, when I started to realize the effort it takes to make something like this happen, I was in shock! I have this thing where I get an idea and then, without questioning myself or my team, I start … only later to realize how much work it's going to be. But that is my weakness and my strength.

Where did your interest in street culture come from? From skateboarding. To this day it's my biggest interest, even though I only skate a couple of times a year now. It's what linked me to other cultures associated with street culture.

Who inspired you when it came to building a label and creating an atmosphere? So many people … not only from fashion. I'm really inspired by Jeff Koons's 'factory' and how he creates his projects. He and his team invent many of the colours and techniques that they use. A lot of his art seems simple and childish at first, but when you look into how it's made it's in a league of its own. I also like many of the newer American menswear designers, like Adam Kimmel, Thom Browne, Humberto Leon, Carol Lim, etc. They understand the art of balancing the classic, fun and wearable with story-telling. Lars Von Trier is also a great inspiration when it comes to atmosphere. I could go on forever…

Business-wise, you must have had someone who guided you in the right direction, because running a business in Denmark or anywhere is not that easy, what with all the regulations… I've had my guides, but for the past few years my business partner Jacob Kampp Berliner and I have run the company together. It's meant a lot for there to be two of us. I would never have been where I am today without Jacob and the rest of our team.

You really hit the right market at the right time. Was it a conscious decision, or something that just happened? I guess it was a conscious decision that just happened. You can do so much but never know the future.

Tell me about your first show and how it came about. I remember we were playing football in the courtyard of our old office, and I said, 'What the hell, let's do a show.' We rented a theatre for the location and I had no idea how the model world worked, so I just had homeboys modelling. I think seventy people showed up and we had nine outfits – a very home-made style – but it worked out and here we are, ten shows later. Today homeboys modelling is very rare and we have a few more outfits. I have great memories, though, of the shows we've done, even the ones that were terrible!

You have no formal training in design, which I think is a good thing, because often when people get out of

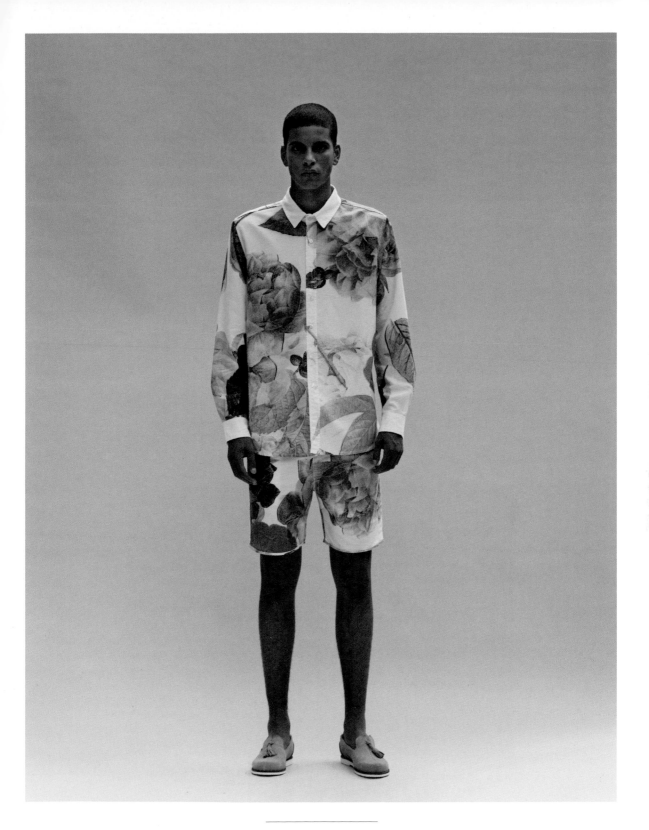

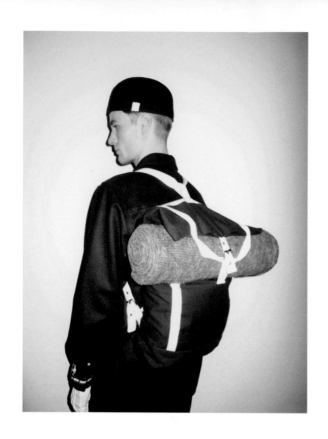

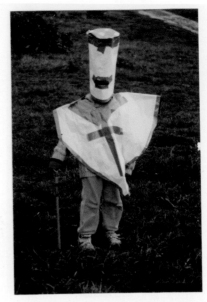

WE ~~WILL~~ NOT ADVERTISE...NEVER!

— S.ADLER

SOULLAND

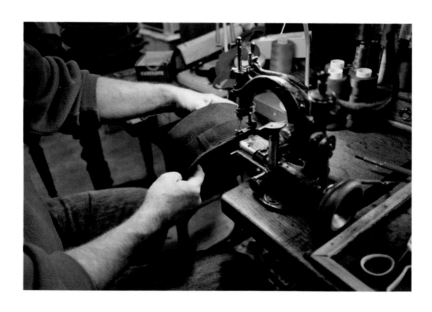

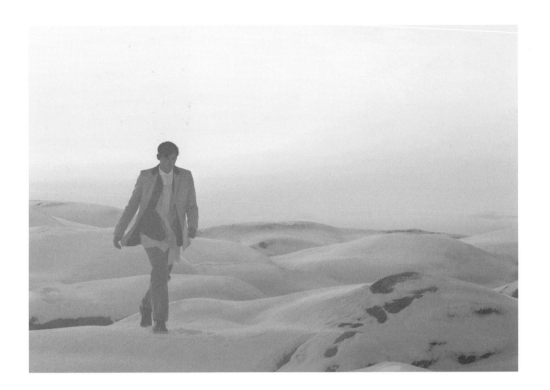

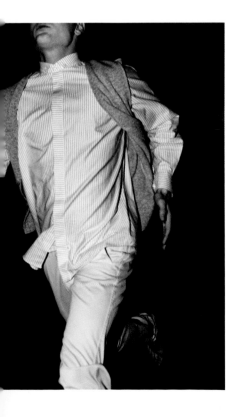

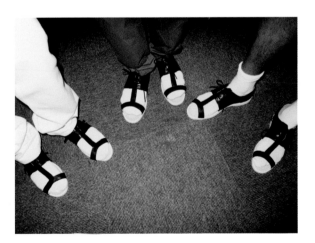

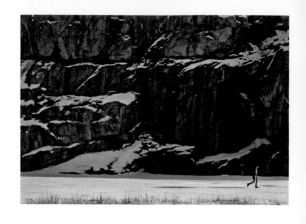

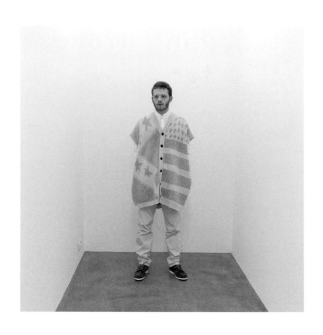

'I constantly get ideas
and I act on them
right away'

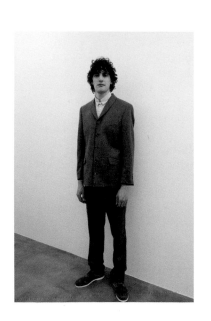

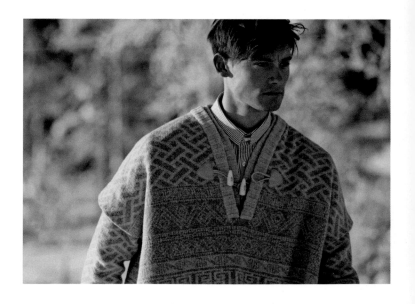

'No schooling means you can never go more wrong than do everything wrong, which is not so bad after all'

ON FASHION EDUCATION

design schools it's like a factory and they come out ready-made but with no idea of what they want. Did you apply anywhere ever? Never. No schooling means you can never go more wrong than do everything wrong, which is not so bad after all.

Tell me about your time in Paris and why you decided to go there. Copenhagen was growing more slowly than I was. I needed a break. I only spent half a year in Paris, but it made me remember what is so fantastic about Copenhagen. Paris is an amazing city, and there are very important things going on when it comes to fashion, but the problem is that there's not very much space for new talent. If you look at New York, Berlin or London, new creative forces are constantly breaking through. You never see that in Paris, and I realized when I lived there that the system is very old in a way. I still look back fondly on the time I spent there, and it's still the most important city for us when it comes to sales. You don't have any other men's fashion week with that level of international press and buyers.

You have been involved with Topman and Goodhood, and you have your collection on Opening Ceremony's website. How did those collaborations happen? Yes, we worked with Topman and we sell to Opening Ceremony in New York and Los Angeles. We also sell our collection to some of the best stores in Europe, such as Colette, Hunting And Collection, Soto, Super A Market, etc. It's super nice to sell to such great stores, and in a way it's the medal for all the hard work. For the last few years we've also been active at the

fashion weeks in New York, Paris, Berlin and Copenhagen, and most of our connections have been made during those very important weeks. But everything takes a lot of time.

Where do you produce your garments? Portugal and Denmark.

Where do you generally look for inspiration? It really varies. It's often a culture or a story that's very specific to a country. In some ways you can say I'm taking a world tour with my collections.

There are some interesting brands coming out of Scandinavia, with the same aesthetics. Why do you think this style fits into the Scandinavian market and also captures the interest of other countries? The answer is simple: it's simple.

You have also collaborated on a few video projects and worked as a stylist on shoots. Where does this interest come from? I just constantly get ideas and I act on them right away. I'm very interested in video and wish I had more time to work with it. Maybe in the future… I like styling my own collections, but to do editorials for other things and publications is boring. Too much in the way of logistics!

I definitely agree that the logistics when styling are insane! What do you see yourself doing in the future? The same thing as now, just bigger, better and more refined.

SPON DIOGO

THE AESTHETICS OF CREATIVE COUPLE MIA SPON AND RUI DIOGO ARE
SUPER-SHARP YET THE PAIR STILL FEEL AS IF THEY'VE JUST STARTED OUT. BASED IN BERLIN,
THEY COMBINE TAILORING AND FINE ARTS IN A MINIMALIST APPROACH, WITH SEASONAL
SHOWS IN COPENHAGEN AND PRESENTATIONS IN PARIS AND BERLIN. AS WINNERS
OF THE 2012 MAX FACTOR 'NEW TALENT' AWARD, THEY WERE GIVEN
THEIR OWN SHOW DURING COPENHAGEN FASHION WEEK.

Rui, you have done so well since you started in 2008. Everything has gone really fast. How do you keep on track when there is such a frenzy around you? We don't feel things really have gone that fast. When we presented the very first season in August 2008, we decided not to rush into cooperation with either sales agents or press agents. We took our time to try and figure out exactly what we wanted to do and how to approach the market. Over time we've worked with different agents, both sales and press. This is a very slow and expensive way of building a label, but we feel in contact with every single decision we've made.

If you had to explain the Spon Diogo universe to someone who had never seen your work before, what would you tell them? Our main focus has always been the body, along with the movement of fabric on it. Tailoring and fabric play a vital role, often more than colour.

You seem to complement each other so well. I can imagine Mia perfecting everything and you taking care of business, ideas and PR. It is not that often you meet people who have such a balanced relationship. We do complement each other very well, but not necessarily in the way described. We're still a very small team. When we're designing and developing the collections, it's a 100% joint effort. We still draw on each other's drawings. Mia is in charge of the atelier and I mostly handle out-of-house sampling and production as well as press and photo shoots.

When and why did you decide, OK, there's nothing out there like this, we need to start our own brand? We met in 2004 (it was love at first kiss) and some time after

that we starting working together on miscellaneous projects, including collections for men and women, knitwear and suiting for local Danish companies. In working together we grew a real liking and shared a view on how to approach the various processes alongside the outcome. Spon Diogo felt as if it was bound to come into existence sooner or later.

Why did you choose to be based in Berlin? Your design seems to have this fine balance of structured lines and delicate details. I imagine you in between New York and Paris. It is actually very hard to place you (which I don't like to do anyway). Berlin obviously has a fantastic art and music scene, but it's also probably the most diverse city I can think of. It holds so many facets and surprises. It is, however, very difficult to work from, as it has no fashion industry. We will most probably move to Paris eventually and set up a studio there.

Where does your inspiration come from? What magazines, films, cities, people inspire you? Our previous collections were very thematically/conceptually designed. They followed a rigorous recipe from theme to research, drawing, selection and lastly development. Now development happens a lot more randomly and the collections are far more mood-based. Influences or inspirations tend to creep up on us or are drawn from our historical repertoire. We are both film buffs, but for inspiration I can't point to any one film in particular.

Can you describe your customer? Previously our starting ground was quite a strict industrial minimalism, but since AW11/12 we've been working on softening the overall expression. One now sees perhaps a softer woman. She is still very

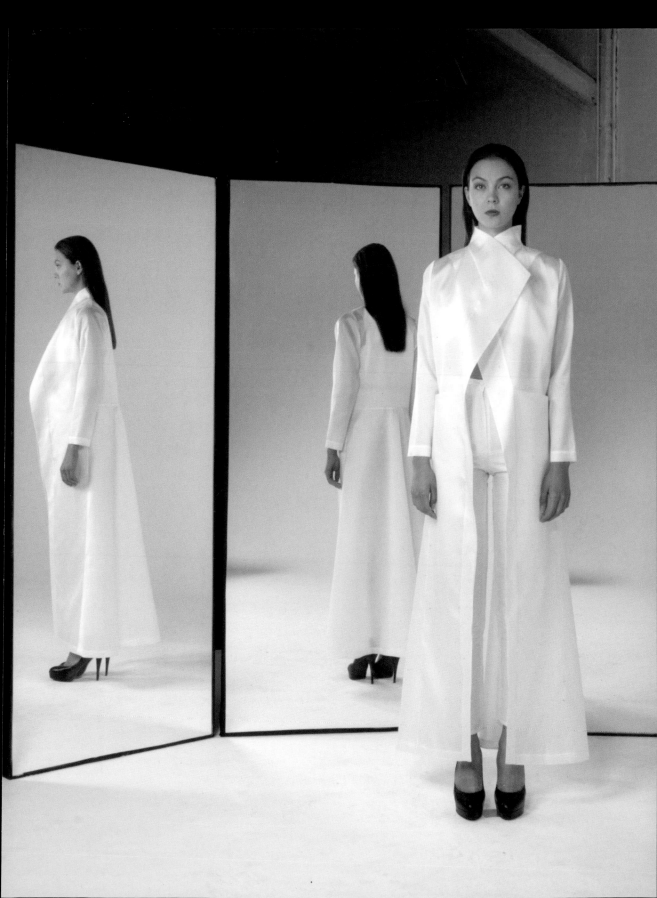

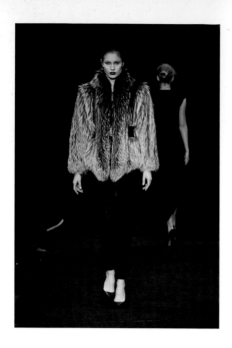

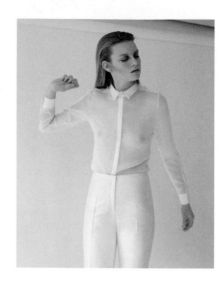

much an urban character and the setting is still a city. She enjoys the better things in life, she will do anything for love, and she is not afraid to go over the top.

For the AW11 collection you had a fur collaboration with Saga Furs. Is that something you plan on expanding in the future? Yes, very much so. We love it! We learned a lot about animals and the vast range of techniques out there. That season also saw a collaboration with a Copenhagen-based corset maker. We also learned a great deal with him. It was enriching to step out of our comfort zone and learn new techniques and crafts. We would love to develop a small range of fur pieces for each collection, also for summer, and that's what we plan on doing.

What is your design process and where is everything produced or manufactured? It's really a very fluid process. Themes usually grow out of the previous collection and are developed further or commented upon. We have discussions for a long period before making a single stroke on paper. Then the drawing and range-planning starts and we select the direction we want to proceed with. We develop only the more complex pieces in our atelier – the ones that need to be tried over and over again. All the sampling and production we place in Europe. Suiting and coats are in Portugal and Italy; all the leatherwork we place in Turkey; and some of the easier dresses, shirts and jackets are developed and produced in Lithuania and Romania.

Do you see yourself also creating shoes, handbags, etc., or collaborating with any brand? Yes, definitely. Shoes and accessories are important for the collection. For the AW12/13 collection, we made a small range of jewelry, and we want to expand into shoes and bags as soon as possible.

Where do you wish to see your brand in the future? It's been our wish from the beginning to create a full label.

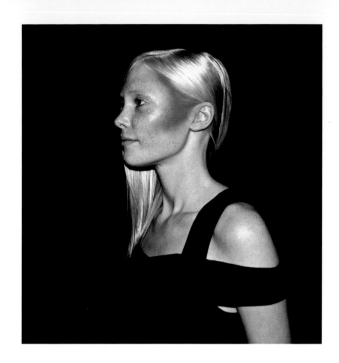

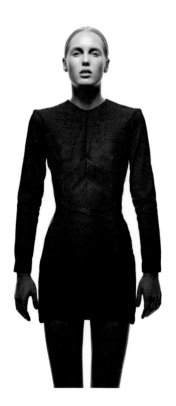

Below: Designers
Mia Spon and Rui Diogo.

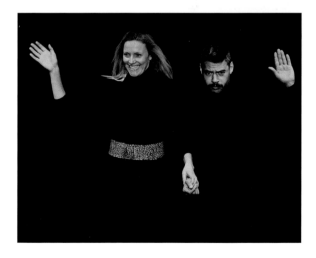

STINE GOYA

THIS DANISH DESIGNER WITH A BACKGROUND AT CENTRAL SAINT MARTINS AND CAREER EXPERIENCE AS A FASHION EDITOR MADE A NAME FOR HERSELF MODELLING FOR KARL LAGERFELD. TODAY SHE RUNS A SUCCESSFUL BRAND, WHICH HAS WON MANY AWARDS, PERHAPS DUE TO HER FOCUS ON A PASTEL PALETTE, THE FEMININE TOUCH AND A BIT OF HELP FROM HER FRIENDS.

Tell me about the beginning of your brand. It all started when I finished my education at Central Saint Martins. I felt I had the energy, and I had an idea of making a unique design and brand built on my own prints, a delicate palette of different but coherent colours, and nice feminine design details with my edge on them. Like everybody else I started with nothing but, thanks to a lot of work, friends and a little bit of luck, I think we have passed the first level of building a brand. Today we have a very good platform to develop the company even further, and that is very exciting.

You were working as the fashion editor at _Cover_ magazine. Did you get tired of styling and communicating design and feel the urge to do your own? I really enjoyed my job and time together with _Cover_. It's a great magazine and a good place to work. But, as I said, I had a strong desire for making my own design and brand.

Tell me what Central Saint Martins was like for you. That is where it all started – my skills as a designer, my first inspirations and so on. Also my teachers and tutors meant a lot to me.

Print is your main thing. How come? I was just very fascinated by the possibility of making my own expressions working with prints, and then I enjoyed the process of making the prints so much. I realized that it was an obvious way of creating something unique and expressive.

How do you feel that you are influencing the direction of Scandinavian design? It's difficult for me to answer that question. I think you have to ask somebody else … but of course I'm interested in hearing the answer!

You have won several awards for your design. What makes it so popular, do you think? I don't know for sure, but I have the feeling that women like it because it's personal, unique and at the same time elegant and feminine. Then I also work hard on developing my design but importantly within the frame of the brand, style and history that I've already created. I think and hope that customers can understand and identify with the design and history.

You tend to work in the same colours, often pastels. What attracts you to those colours? For me these colours suit almost every woman – that's why! The colours are soft and delicate, and you can mix them in so many different ways and still they suit each other.

When you started out, did you begin with a smaller collection? How did you finance the start-up, which can be very costly? I started slowly and got a lot of help from good friends, but also had a little financial help.

How come you chose to be located in Denmark? That was easier because it's where I had my roots, my network and back-up, in many ways.

Where do you produce your garments? Is anything made in Scandinavia? It's all produced outside of Scandinavia, in almost ten different countries.

What are you currently working on? We're selling our first pre-spring collection. Luckily our customers seem to like it. Next I have to finish the SS collection, then I have to work on the AW collection, then after that I have to start up the pre-autumn collection…

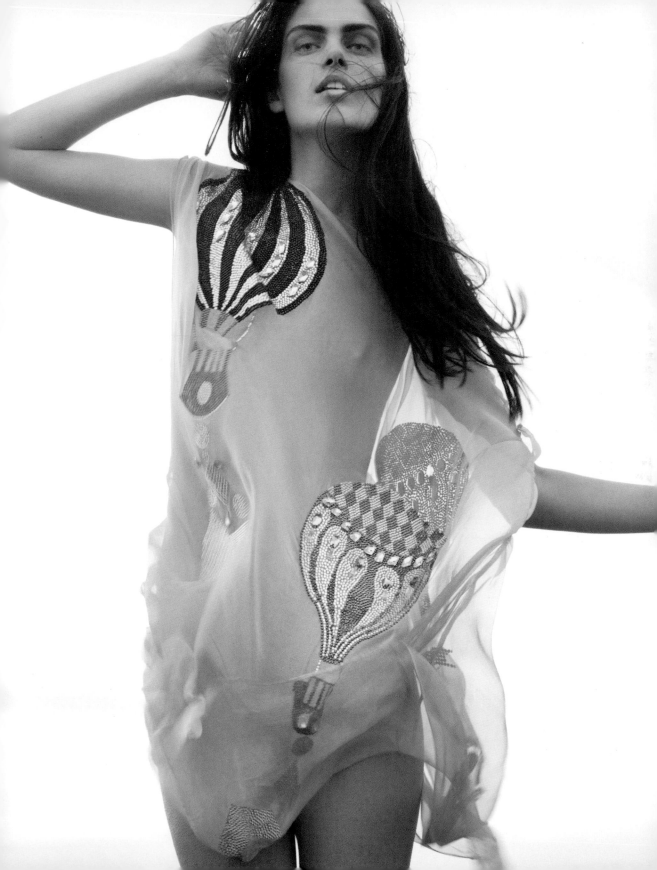

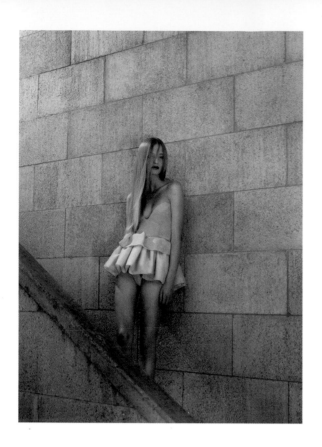

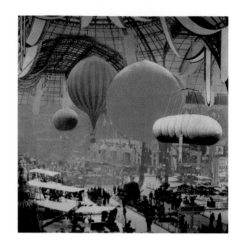

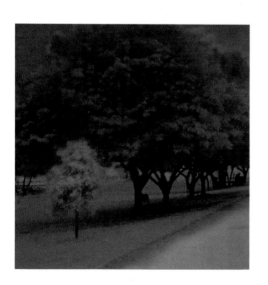

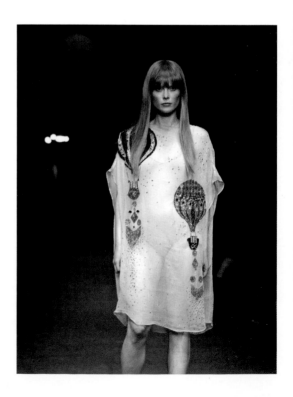

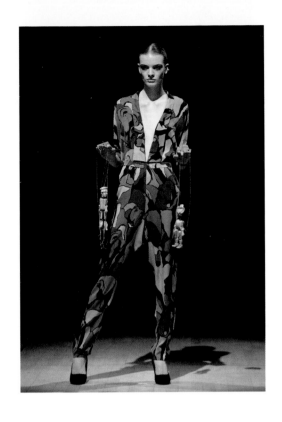

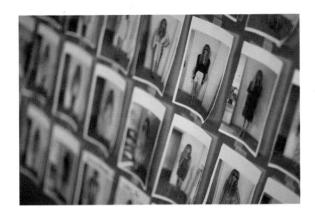

Below: Designer Stine Goya
on the runway.

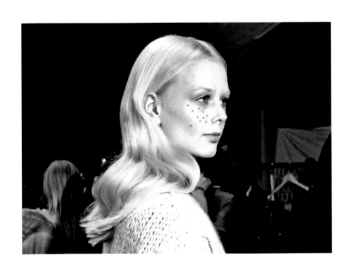

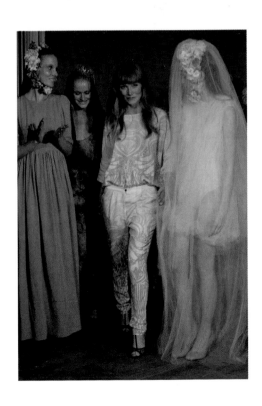

TIGER OF SWEDEN

THIS IMPRESSIVE COMPANY DATES BACK MORE THAN 100 YEARS, TO A TIME WHEN TAILORING WAS TRADITIONAL. THE BRAND HAS MOVED EXTREMELY FAST IN RECENT YEARS, WITH MULTIPLE OWN-BRAND STORES AND OVER 1,200 RETAILERS WORLDWIDE. THE COMPANY PHILOSOPHY IS TO CREATE A NEW INTERPRETATION OF WELL-TAILORED SCANDINAVIAN FASHION WITH A CHARACTER OF ITS OWN.

Tiger of Sweden is a pretty old brand, dating from 1903. Per [Håkans], as Marketing Director, can you tell me about its beginnings? Tiger of Sweden started out as a gentleman's brand for old farts with funny hats in a small town in Sweden! But Marcus Schwartzman and his partner Hjalmar Nordström founded the company on the basis of one great idea. They would turn the traditional working methods of the tailor upside down, in that they would go to customers instead of sitting in the shop and waiting for customers to come to them.

What has been the key to the company's success? Everything comes down to a sharp concept and brand DNA. It's not as if the world has a shortage of brands, so you really have to be different. The suit, for example, has been done a thousand times, so it's not about reinventing the wheel but more about repackaging the wheel. You have to find your brand identity; find out what works and stay true to it. We have our foundation in a strong confection tradition and solid tailoring skills refined for over a hundred years. In 1993 our brand was repositioned with a clear vision of 'taking the suit out of the bank and into the street'. Since then, we've gone from being a tailoring brand for gentlemen to being an international design brand, including men's, women's and jeans collections with a wide range of shoes and accessories. For us, it's important constantly to challenge the fashion scene, and we work in close collaboration with the best fabric mills available, developing our own fabric designs that create the brand's uniqueness.

Every season you present your collection during Stockholm Fashion Week. Have you presented anywhere else? Do you present at any international fairs? We haven't done shows elsewhere, but it shouldn't be a surprise if we do so in the future. We are at 'Bread & Butter' in Berlin and at the 'Fashion Fair' in Copenhagen.

What are your main markets and who are your main customers? Tiger of Sweden attracts a creative citizen, who moves effortlessly between different cosmopolitan environments; an independent individual, who loves a clean, well-fitted, tailored cut, with high quality and a modern Scandinavian attitude. Today we have Tiger of Sweden shops in Sweden, Denmark, Norway, Finland, Germany, Canada and South Africa, our own webshop and a total of 1,200 retailers spread over 18 countries on three continents. Having that said, it's quite fascinating that we meet the same kind of customer in all our markets.

Is everything made in Sweden in your design studio and then sent off to the factory, or how do you work? All our products are designed in Stockholm, and all our ready-to-wear suits and jackets are produced in Europe using European fabrics, mainly Italian.

Who developed the visual aspect of your brand – the campaigns and website? Nowadays we develop and create the majority ourselves.

What are you inspired by when you design? Our mantra is: what would we wear? For us, tailoring is about fit, about accentuating the body. We take the tailored look, give it a twist and make a fashion statement. For us, the suit is something you can wear to work, to the bar across the street, or even to the nightclub, and still look sharp. Tiger of Sweden's updated definition of well-tailored fashion paired with Scandinavian design values creates a clean cut that we like to play with; something that we define as 'laid-back luxury'. Classic cuts with non-

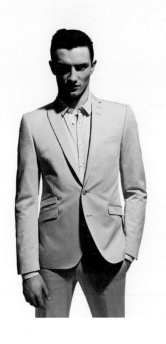

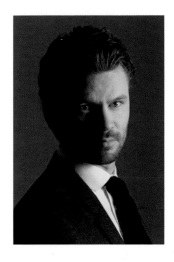

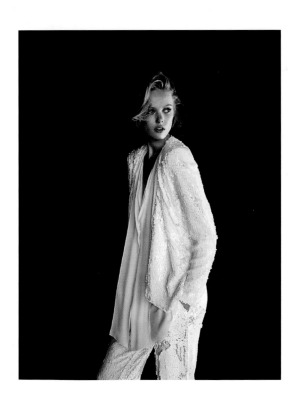

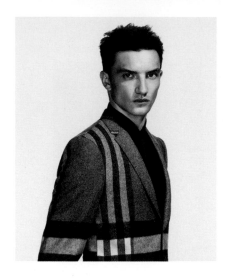

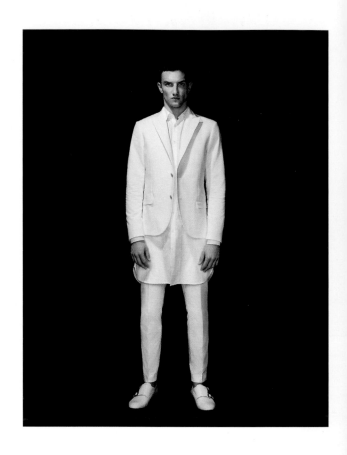

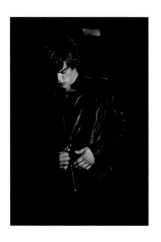

classic materials and patterns, and vice versa. We call it 'A Different Cut'. It's a concept that goes beyond what you can accomplish with scissors, fabrics, thread and stitches and extends into a brand philosophy.

What does it mean for you to be a Swedish design brand? Tiger of Sweden was born with innovation and curiosity woven into its DNA spiral. This is our greatest strength and is something we will never give up. But it places enormous demands – not just on the products and our brand but also on us as a company. Our organization and our processes must continually develop at the same rate as our ambitions. In this context, 'A Different Cut' is more important now than ever before. Every day, we will wake up and create a new interpretation of well-tailored Scandinavian fashion with a character of its own. In the international arena, Tiger of Sweden is associated with its own on-target look – minimalistic, with a modern cut; affordable luxury in its purest form. But the international fashion scene always presents completely new challenges, which is exactly what drives us to carry on.

'Find your brand identity, find out what works and stay true to it'

ON IDENTITY

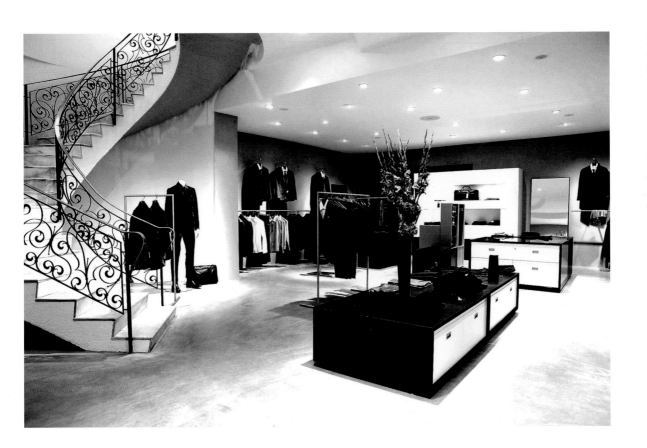

VERONICA B. VALLENES

THIS PRIZE-WINNING NORWEGIAN DESIGNER IS BASED IN COPENHAGEN.
HER COLLECTIONS HAVE GAINED INTERNATIONAL RECOGNITION IN MAGAZINES
SUCH AS DAZED & CONFUSED, POP, PIG, FALLEN AND SMUG. SHE HAS ALSO WON
THE PRESTIGIOUS DANISH MAX FACTOR 'NEW TALENT' AWARD, WHICH
INCLUDED A SHOW AT COPENHAGEN CITY HALL.

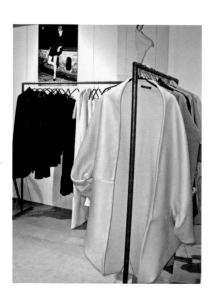

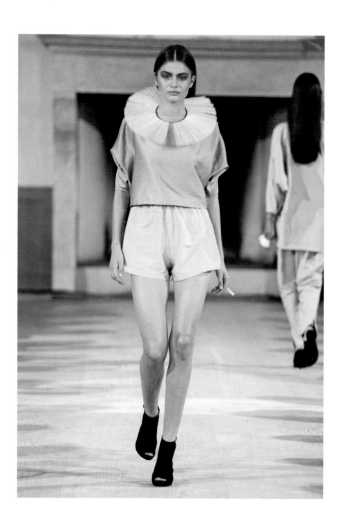

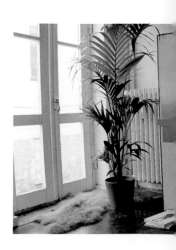

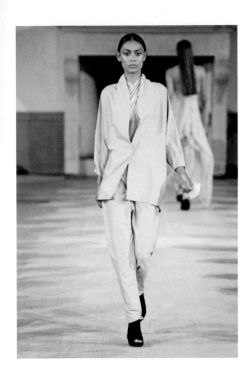

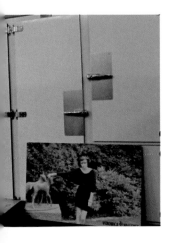

Tell me about your upbringing in Norway. Did you study fashion there? I grew up in the south, by the sea, in quite a small place, where I spent a lot of my time dreaming, drawing, sewing, making sculptures, and reading art books and old fashion magazines. I had a style of my own. When I was 15, I wore men's suits and smoked cigarettes with a silver cigarette holder, and that wasn't so usual in a small town! But we had a big music festival, where artists like David Bowie, Björk, Nick Cave and Beck came to play. It was always the highlight of the year, and the town became more exotic. I started sewing when I was 12, and after high school I went to the faculty of Fashion and Costume Design at the National College of Art and Design in Oslo.

Does any of that transfer into your design today? I think you can see the Scandinavian minimalism in my design, combined with the dream of exotic, sensual places. Contact with nature has also always been a big part of my life, but I can't tell if you can see that in my design.

You don't have as many fashion designers in Norway as Denmark or Sweden. Why do you think that is? No, we don't, and I think that's sad. I think some of the designers are either too commercial or too experimental, but there are a lot of talents there so I hope that we'll see a change, and that the Norwegian government will make an effort and support designers so that Norway can build up its own design identity.

Why did you choose Copenhagen Fashion Week to present your collection, rather than the Norwegian fashion week? It's a totally different thing. The fashion week in Norway doesn't attract buyers or international press (in fact, it barely attracts national press) in the same way as Copenhagen Fashion Week does. It has really helped my career, both nationally and internationally, to present in Copenhagen.

You are now based in Copenhagen. What made you move? I've always loved the atmosphere, and I understood quite early that if I was going to establish myself in the fashion industry I had to move away from Norway.

Do you run a small team? How do you manage to construct each collection? It's a very small team, so the days are long, but we're planning to expand very soon. I love the process of making the collections and sewing the first sample, and I learn a lot being part of every process, but the business side takes way too much time, so I'm really looking forward to having a bigger team.

'I think you can see the Scandinavian minimalism in my design, combined with the dream of exotic, sensual places'

ON IDENTITY

You have received some great awards. What do you think makes your design something that people notice and appreciate? I think it must be the combination of laid-back elegance and edge. Some of the silhouettes are innovative but still wearable and flattering for the female body, and the garments are made with good materials.

You have also been featured already in *Vogue*, *Wallpaper* and *Vanity Fair*, and on national TV. That happened quite fast, didn't it, or have you been working on it for a long time? I'm incredibly happy about it. The years between my graduation and my breakthrough, if you can call it that, were extremely hard. I was working night and day, and I didn't have any money or recognition, just a very big passion and a dream. There were so many times I thought I couldn't go on, it was too humiliating, and I had to find something else to do, but my passion was too strong to let go. And suddenly things started to happen, and I can't tell you how much it means to me.

How do you organize your team? Is your daily life all about work? Yes, I don't have much of a social life. Luckily I have a patient boyfriend, and the people I work with are fantastic.

What is your design style inspired by? It's vintage references combined with contemporary references. It's draped silhouettes combined with straight lines; no unnecessary details.

Your fabrics seems to be very delicate and luxurious. Is that something you focus on with subtle colours rather than bold statements? Yes, I love working with delicate, good-quality fabric – the feeling you get when you wear one, the way it moves around the body. I get a lot of my ideas when I hold a fabric and use the way it falls. My style is more relaxed and my focus is on the person that will be wearing it. I want them to feel comfortable, beautiful and cool. For my style that is more important, but I love watching other designers make bold statements.

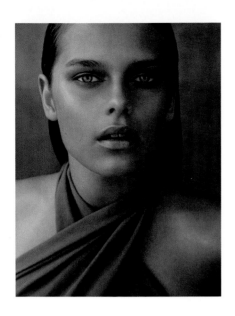

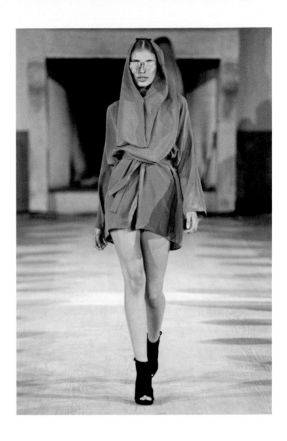

'Draped silhouettes
combined with straight lines;
no unnecessary details'

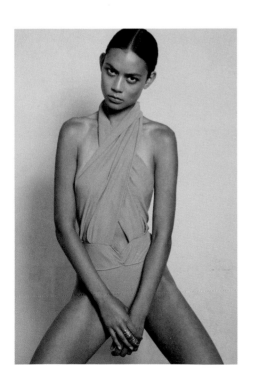

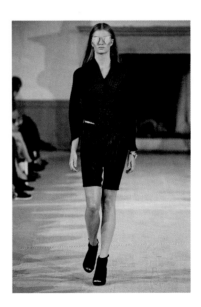

VILSBØL DE ARCE

TWO FRIENDS FROM DESIGN SCHOOL – PRISCA VILSBØL AND PIA DE ARCE –
MET WITH A COMMON AMBITION AND A DRIVE TO EXCEL AND DIFFER FROM THE REST.
THEY HAVE MANAGED TO PRODUCE COLLECTIONS WITHOUT SUCCUMBING TO MASS-MARKET
COMMERCIALISM. LIVING IN THEIR OWN CREATIVE UNIVERSE, FOLDING PAPER AND
MOULDING CLAY TO FIND NEW SHAPES, THEY HAVE SUCCEEDED IN DRESSING
STARS SUCH AS LADY GAGA, PEACHES AND NATALIE PORTMAN.

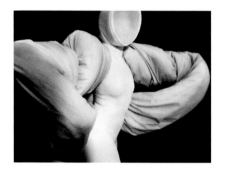

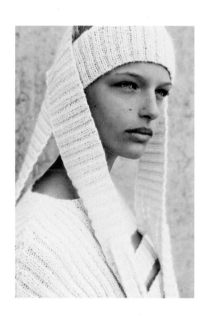

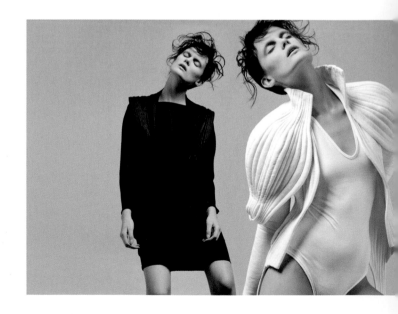

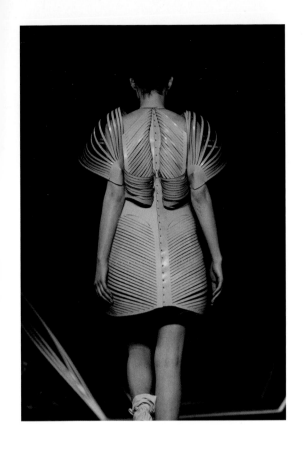

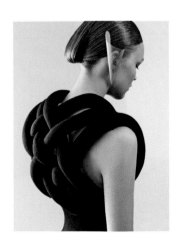

Tell me about your universe. We have always been fascinated by the concept of armour – clothing that gives the wearer strength and protection, while also sending a strong message to impress the adversary. By putting it on, your whole body language changes. Your shoulders straighten, you feel taller; it gives you an upright, dignified posture. It is this feeling we would like to give our wearers.

Where did you both grow up, and when did you start working together? Both of us have travelled a lot ever since we were very young. Pia's parents are Chilean and, though she was born and schooled in Denmark, she travelled a lot to South America and Europe as a child, then after high school she spent a couple of years working abroad before returning to Copenhagen. Prisca was born in Paris to French-Danish parents, and spent seven years living in South East Asia before graduating high school in France and moving to Copenhagen in 2000. We met in Copenhagen on a private two-year fashion course. While the school in itself was not a very ambitious one, we recognized in each other a similar drive, and therefore encouraged each other to go further. After graduation in 2002, we immediately decided to start a company together, although at the time we had little idea of what that meant. We had to start from scratch with everything, from design process to tax form, and most of what we know today comes from the experiments made as partners in a newly founded company. The current company, Vilsbøl de Arce, was founded in 2007.

What sort of research or study do you do before designing a collection? We tend to start every collection by exploring a subject outside the realm of fashion, the idea being that you can make a collection out of anything and, if you get fascinated enough, you can make it into a consistent concept. Then the process of investigation starts. Once the rules are there, we can start exploring, twisting, pulling and cutting to see what this particular concept is capable of. For example, the urge to experiment with volumes makes us spend innumerable hours folding strips or squares of paper, searching for new shapes to test on the body. Growing up in the present era of extreme production and consumption, we feel the need to justify the existence of each piece of clothing, and this in-depth work process allows us to do so.

Your collections have often generated their own art projects. Why is this important to you? It's actually the other way around. The first pieces of each collection are created without commercial or wearable considerations or limitations, and we always strive to start out a process with total freedom

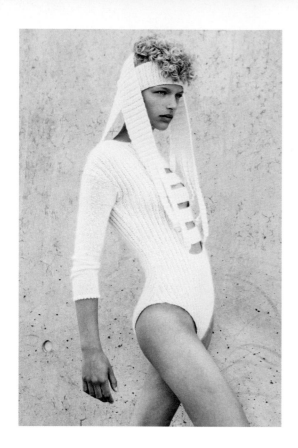

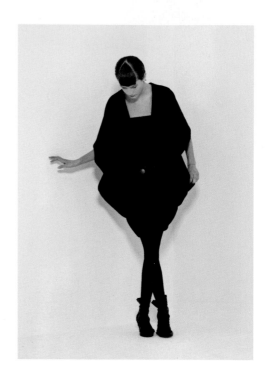

of expression. This is where the showpieces and art projects have developed. It's a way of expanding our minds before focusing on a collection, and a way to find original and challenging shapes, which can then be translated into ready-to-wear pieces.

What is the strangest material you've ever worked with? We will work with just about anything during the design process. Mock-ups are made with paper, plastic, clay, cement, foam, staples, rope; you name it! But when it comes to the final clothing, we try to translate the effect into comfortable, preferably natural materials.

You were 'discovered' abroad because Lady Gaga wore one of your bodies. How did that happen, and has it had an impact on the brand? We met a lot of amazing people who saw potential in our designs right from the beginning. Samuel Drira and Sybille Walter from *Encens* magazine introduced us to the Parisian press agency Cristofolipress, who

took our brand from the second collection and really pushed our designs in Paris and abroad. Thanks to them, stars like Lady Gaga, Peaches, Rihanna, Fischerspooner, Natalie Portman and others were seen in our designs. There is no doubt that it's these events that gave the brand its international recognition, as well as giving us the spotlight for the 'Talent of the Year' award, which we won at the Danish Fashion Awards 2010.

What is the future for the brand? Since the beginning we have striven to give ourselves pure creative freedom, preferring to avoid the fleeting trends and overproduction so common in the fashion industry. The company has now grown to be a full-blown business, following the seasonal sales, etc., but the essence is still the same – to have a company structure that allows research and unbridled creativity as well as really good products. We keep optimizing to reach that goal, and are now looking forward to having new partners in the company who can help take Vilsbøl de Arce to the next level.

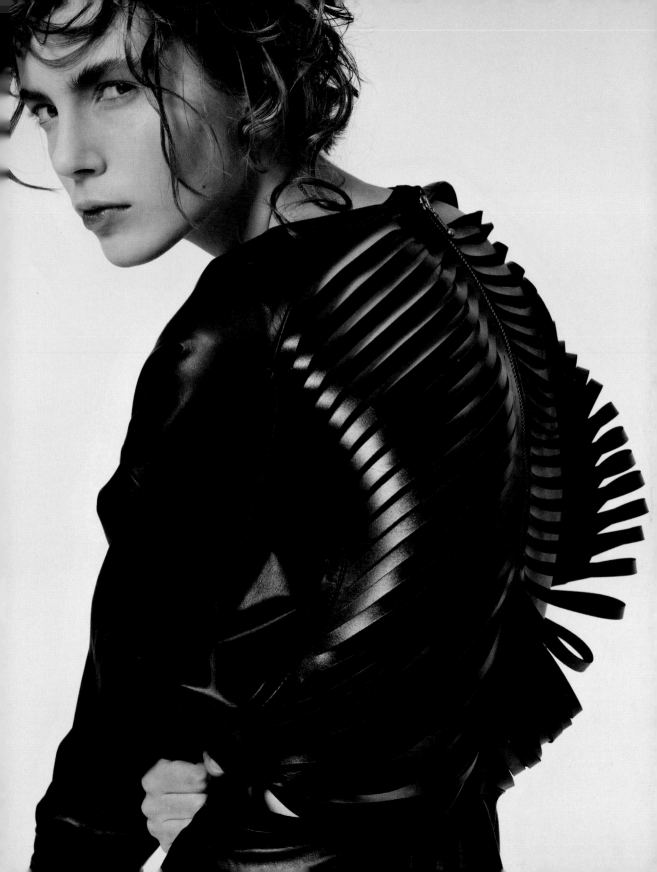

WEEKDAY

FROM SECOND-HAND TO HIGH STREET: WHAT STARTED OUT
AS A SMALL VINTAGE SHOP IN A STOCKHOLM SUBURB – FOUNDED BY
FOUR FRIENDS, INCLUDING ÖRJAN ANDERSSON AND ADAM FRIBERG – BECAME
THE CELEBRATED WEEKDAY. AFTER JOINING FORCES WITH H&M, THE COMPANY
HAS OPENED STORES IN DENMARK, NORWAY, FINLAND AND GERMANY,
AND IS SET TO CONQUER THE WORLD.

The original second-hand shop was called Weekend because it was only open on Saturdays and Sundays. Located far from Stockholm's main shopping streets, it nonetheless stocked a great selection of vintage garments. The founders, together with entrepreneur Lasse Karlsson, decided to open a larger shop in a more central location. This new store was open every day and carried a mix of high fashion, smaller independent labels and vintage clothing. When it turned out that denim was expensive, Örjan Andersson launched the first Cheap Monday tight jeans, which were an immediate success. In 2008, the company teamed up with the H&M Group and has since expanded to Denmark, Norway, Finland and Germany, and is intent on capturing the world.

Along with Weekday's bold ideas comes a humble attitude, which they believe has been their way forward. Their desire is to offer creative fashion at affordable prices. The six brands comprising the Weekday store experience are Cheap Monday (the limited range of tight jeans with characteristic skull logo has expanded to a line of fashion garments for men and women), Weekday Vintage (continuing Weekend's original concept but always with a view to complimenting contemporary outfits), Weekday Collaboration (limited editions created with invited designers), Weekday Storemade (unique pieces handmade in-store), MTWTFSS Weekday (the in-house brand, including shoes, underwear and accessories) and MTWTFSS Weekday Collection (a tailored, luxury range of updated classics). Each of the stores has a different concept. The Stockholm branch, for example, has sloping floors, tilting mirrors and an 'invisible ghost' effect in the changing rooms. Each store maintains its originality but has a recognizable Weekday touch, which means it doesn't look like any other store.

Every season the company seeks out talents, whether new or established. Collaborators have included Central Saint Martins graduate Peter Jensen (see p. 184), Danish designer Stine Goya (see p. 220), Swedish designer Carin Wester (see p. 56), the acclaimed Belgian Bruno Pieters and the international brand Bless, to name but a few. Weekday also publishes a magazine, often featuring its collaborators alongside interviews with influential figures in fashion. Magazine launches might be celebrated with an in-store party or a happening. But Weekday collaborations encompass a whole universe of creative people, not just fashion designers. Their support of music, art and dance can be seen, for example, in their teaming up with the Royal Swedish Opera.

Like many Scandinavian brands, Weekday is a firm believer in corporate social responsibility. Their objectives are to insist on good working conditions for both staff and suppliers, to respect human rights and to work sustainably. Their products are free from harmful chemicals, they don't use fur or feathers, and they try to minimize wastage. They have also joined the UN Millennium Development Goal of halving poverty by 2015 by engaging in partnerships. Working with the Red Cross, they have created a T-shirt and bag to support efforts to reunite families shattered by war: 100% of the proceeds go to charity.

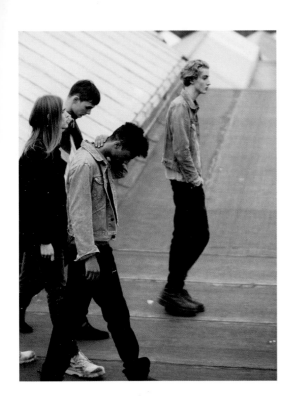

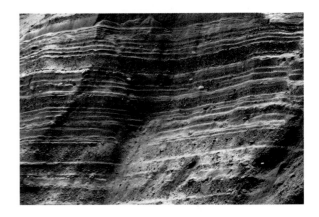

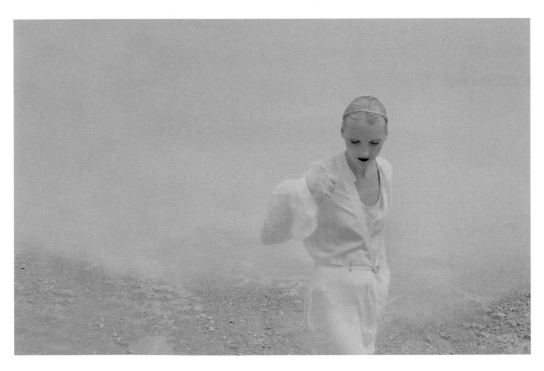

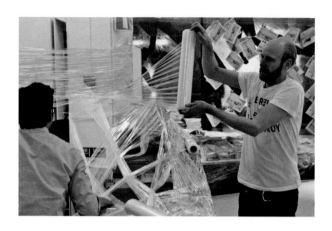

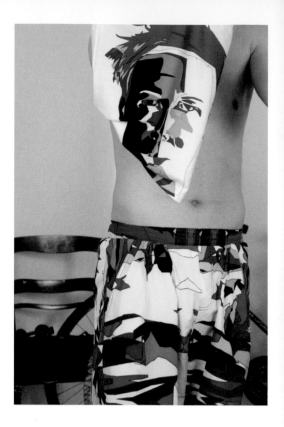

Above: Co-founder Örjan Andersson working on an installation.

Below: An installation by Bless in collaboration with Weekday.

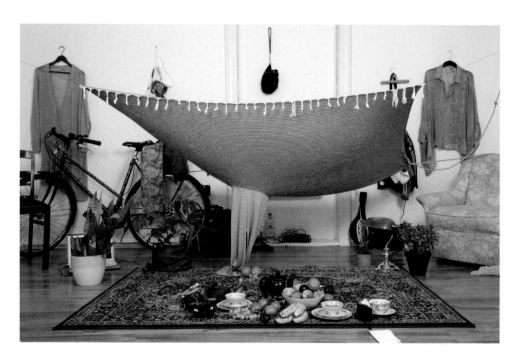

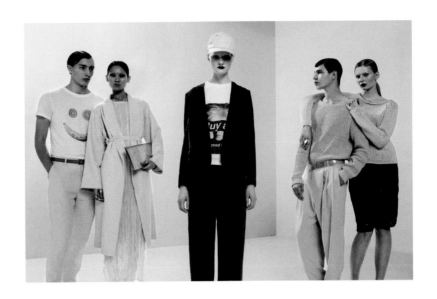

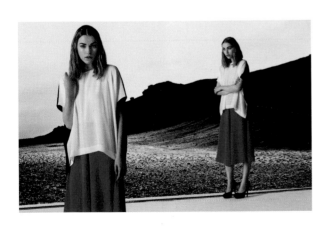

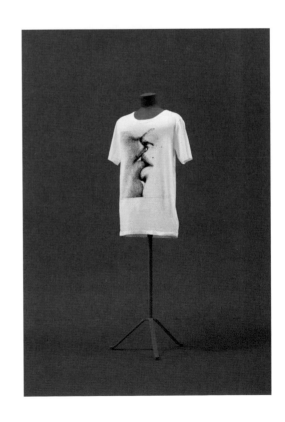

WHYRED

THE SWEDISH INDIE LABEL FOUNDED BY ROLAND HJORT,
LENA PATRIKSSON AND JONAS CLAESSON IS A CONTEMPORARY TAKE ON THE
MUSIC AND ART SCENE. THEIR BEAUTIFUL SHOPS AND CLOTHING, BOTH MINIMALISTIC
AND ATMOSPHERIC, TAKE US TO A STREAMLINED 1960S MOD CULTURE
COMBINED WITH TRADITIONAL SCANDINAVIAN AESTHETICS.

Roland, what is a modernist in your eyes? Someone who likes contemporary art and has a personal view of his/her wardrobe. I see a resemblance of a modernist to an individualist.

When you have done features in magazines or on blogs, there seem to be many references to the 1960s. What draws you to this era? It's not actually the music or style of the 1960s; it's the aesthetics of the Mod culture from that time. 'Clean living under difficult circumstances.' To me, that means a clean Italian suit with a military parka.

How and why did you start Whyred? Whyred was born in 1998 via me, Lena Patriksson and Jonas Claesson. We wanted to start a brand that was made for the observer.

Tell me why you are known as 'the super indie brand'. We celebrate the individualist in all aspects of music, art and personal wardrobe.

Are your garments manufactured in Sweden or mostly abroad, outside of Europe? They're manufactured in Italy, Turkey, Portugal, Romania and China.

How has your brand developed over the years. Have you felt any changes? There has always been a red thread throughout the years. For example, we are still selling the same parka today that we launched in 1999. We have the same ambition and goal today as we had back then.

You judged the competition at the Fresh Fish Fair in Gothenburg consisting of new Swedish talent. Did you see any tendencies in their collections or any movement? No, I didn't really see any tendencies. In fact, I wish I could see more contemporary and daring fashion. I see more of that in the art and music industry today.

Your interests span art and music as well. Did you ever play music or did you want to be an artist but express your vision through fashion? I've never played music but I've always been interested in art. In fact, I'm working on an art project myself. My grandfather was a famous artist and art has always been a big part of my life.

What is your next move? Whyred is working more actively with art and music projects, which have always been important to us. We have several collaborations that we are proud of, and we have more interesting activities ahead!

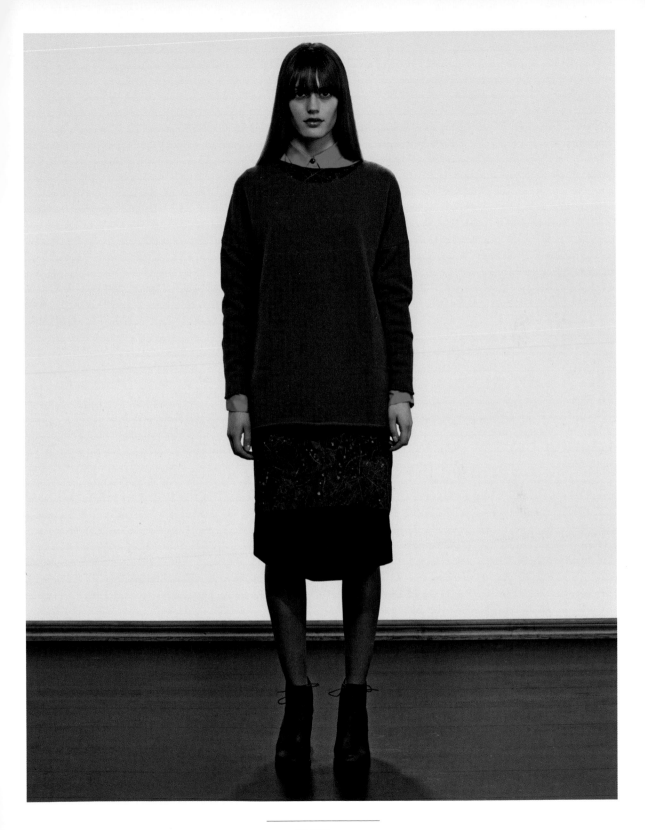

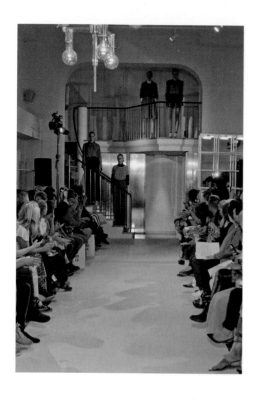

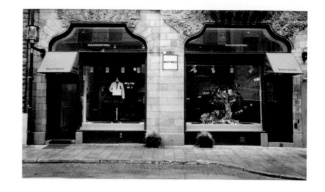

<u>Above:</u> Whyred shop in Stockholm.

<u>Below:</u> Designer Roland Hjort at the finale of a Whyred show in Stockholm

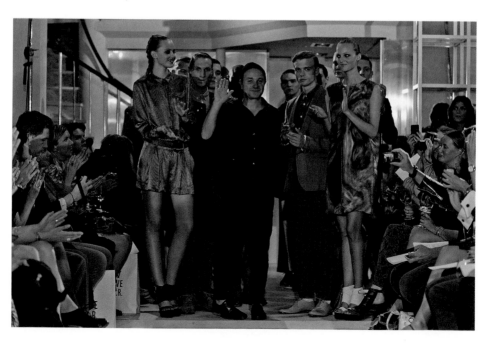

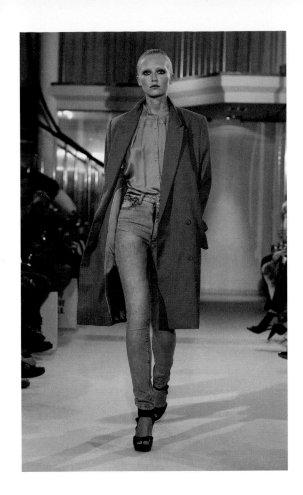

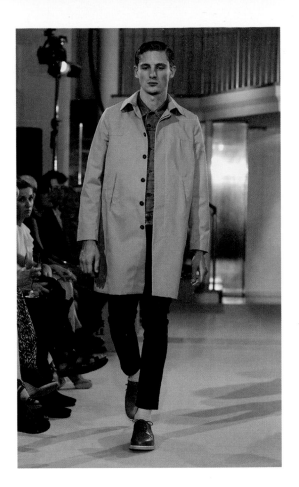

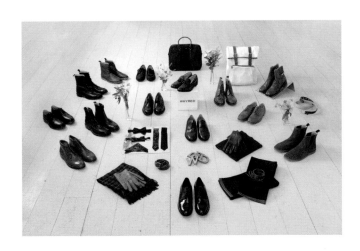

WOOD WOOD

KARL-OSKAR OLSEN AND BRIAN SS JENSEN CAME TOGETHER, ALONG
WITH A FRIEND, TO CREATE ONE OF DENMARK'S COOLEST STREETWEAR BRANDS.
FROM SIMPLE PRINTED T-SHIRTS TO FULL COLLECTIONS IN 4 FLAGSHIP STORES AND SOME
220 SHOPS, AND WITH COLLABORATIONS WITH EVERYONE FROM ADIDAS TO HAPPY
SOCKS, THIS HUGELY POPULAR BRAND HAS BEEN A CONTRIBUTING FACTOR IN THE
SCANDINAVIAN REPUTATION FOR NONCHALANT URBAN COOLNESS.

Karl-Oskar, you do the design for Wood Wood, together with Brian Jensen and womenswear designer Lotte Bank Nielsen. Can you tell me how the brand began? Wood Wood started out doing screenprinted T-shirts in limited editions. Around the millennium a lot of creative people with roots in street culture got involved in making products. This made us realize that we could reach out to a lot of people with our ideas, and we started the brand in the summer of 2002. In the beginning we sold our designs in our own little 20m² basement store in the centre of Copenhagen. We had no plan to what we did; we just did it. But what made us what we are today is that we created everything ourselves, we purchased everything we felt was dope, and we kept moving on to explore new horizons. Around 2006 we decided to make a complete cut-and-sew collection for men and women, and this is now sold in around 220 stores worldwide alongside our flagship stores in Copenhagen, Berlin, Vienna and Aarhus.

Why the name Wood Wood? When we took over our first little store in Krystalgade in Copenhagen, the walls were made of old wood. We talked about calling the store 'Wood'. We really didn't know what to call it, but I'd just seen the movie *Goodfellas* and there's a character called Jimmy Two Times. He always says the last part of a sentence twice, so we called the company 'Wood Wood'. Back then we never thought we would come this far. Perhaps we would have considered the name a bit more if that had been the case!

Do you feel as if you represent Danish style or Scandinavian style in general? We like to think of ourselves as global; we just happen to have a base here in Copenhagen. I guess in some ways you can see or feel the Scandinavian way of thinking about design in terms of aesthetics, materials and structure, which is important, but we always mix our inspiration stories together quite chaotically so they won't become too recognizably Danish or Scandinavian.

Is anything from your collection made in Scandinavia, or is it mostly made abroad? We do produce a small collection of knitwear here in Denmark. It's a factory we've worked with since day one. We had to be competitive on the price and quality so we had to move the rest of our production out.

Tell me about a normal day for you in the office. A normal day is a day where I end up sitting with a lot of stuff that I have to sort out not too late after a deadline! We are based in a five-floor house, where we all do things such as sales, production, logistics, web, design, retail management, etc., so I get to speak to many interesting people all day long.

How are the different roles distributed? As we are growing quite rapidly we need to have a structure and understanding of each other's core areas. In the beginning we tried to do everything ourselves, but now we are taking on more and more people with special qualities to fulfill our goal of becoming the leading brand on the international street fashion scene.

Do you travel to find inspiration, or does it mostly come from the scene around you? We try to travel for inspiration stories, as we always find out about a lot of new things on trips — also against ourselves. It's very healthy to see things from a new perspective.

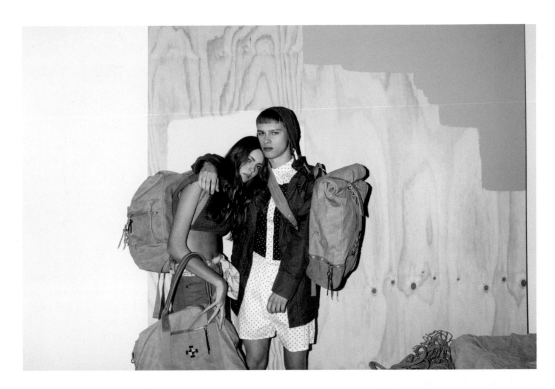

Above: A campaign for
Eastpak vs. Wood Wood.

Below: A 'Brickism'
T-shirt collaboration by
Wood Wood x Colette,
in association with Lego.

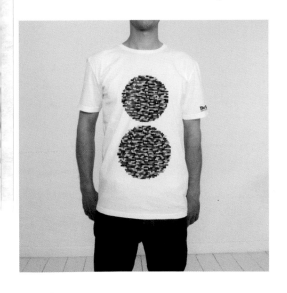

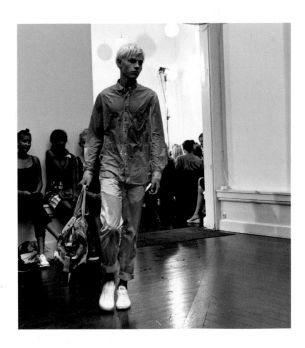

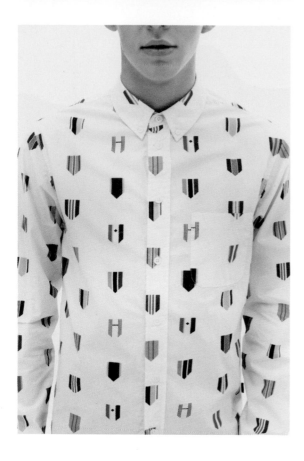

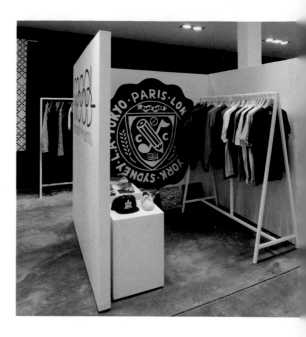

It seems as if many people who used to skate or do graffiti are now creative directors or designers or active in something that's in some way visual but more mass-market. Why do you think that community often moves into fashion? Being in fashion comes very naturally to many of us, as we all purchased a certain style when b-boying, skating or writing. Those cultures were all about style and attitude, and I guess we just took it further by getting involved with this. We still use the strong energy from the street in everything we do.

Tell me about some of your collaborations, because you have had many. How did they happen? Collaborations have been very important for us, as we've used this tool to reach out to people and show what we're about. We've worked with some of the greatest brands in the world, and we've always been urged to use the Wood Wood touch and mentality very specifically incorporated in the products. Wood Wood is also about breaking the rules. We have a motto – 'Not to be trusted' – and by employing this we have the right to go in different directions. That is our core value, and I think that's why all our collaborations have been very successful.

You recently moved into a new space in Copenhagen and it is noticeable that the brand is growing. How have things changed? In growing and opening more stores our next big challenge is how to keep moving in the direction that we still think it's cool to be. Personally I enjoy this challenge, as some things seem easier now than five years ago. With our latest 280m^2 store here in Copenhagen we are able to reach out to many people that are aware of Wood Wood and enjoy our products but would never walk down a small side street to find a store, so in general I think the change is very positive.

What is your next step? The United States is a strong market for us, so expanding there with more shops and two or three flagship stores is the next move.

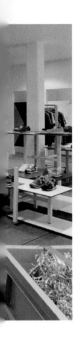

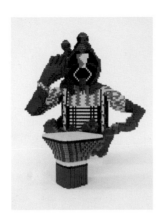

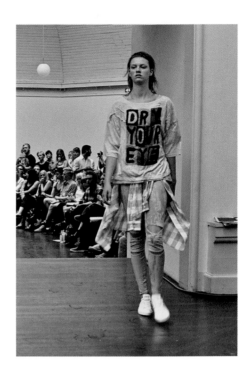

Above: A 'Brickism' Wood Wood
and Lego collaboration, with
artists HuskMitNavn, Delta,
Will Sweeney and So Me.

Left and below:
Shop in Copenhagen.

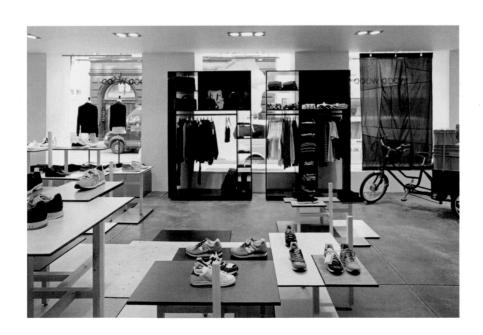

YDE BY OLE YDE

HE IS ONE OF THE DESIGNERS THE SCANDINAVIAN ROYALS AND
OTHER HIGH-END CLIENTELE GO TO WHEN IT COMES TO GETTING WHAT THEY WANT
IN A DRESS. HIS UNIVERSE IS A MIX OF EARLY YVES SAINT LAURENT MEETS MARIE ANTOINETTE,
AND THE 18TH CENTURY JUST SEEMS TO BE FOLLOWING HIM.

You seem to be a bit inspired by Parisian women and the way they dress. Where does your imagining of these chic garments come from? Did you grow up around women like that? Ever since I was a boy, I've been fascinated by stylish, glamorous women. I wasn't necessarily surrounded by that world in real life, only in my imagination and thoughts.

Are there any designers, such as Yves Saint Laurent, that you are inspired by? Yes, the designer that I've always admired the most is Yves Saint Laurent, but I look up to many of the great old ones.

You present your collection in Paris and Copenhagen. Tell me about the differences between the two. Our show in Copenhagen is mostly geared towards our private clients in Scandinavia. Through Paris we can reach a much larger audience.

You moved from Odense in Denmark to Copenhagen to attend design school, but you left short of graduation. How come? My instincts and my dream of designing what I wanted took over. It was beyond me. I thought the timing was right, and and I couldn't wait a day longer.

You won the design prize awarded by the upmarket department store Illum, and you've won several other awards. What do you think makes your designs win? Honesty.

Is everything handmade? If not, how do you go about the production, and where are the fabrics from? We do many one-of-a-kind pieces that require a lot of handwork in our atelier for private clients, but our prêt-à-porter collection is meant to be produced in larger quantities. Our fabrics come mostly from Italy, France and Switzerland.

Who is your YDE Atelier line designed for, and what sort of clients have you had? YDE Atelier caters to women of all ages who want the experience of having their dream dress made for them. These unique pieces may be elegant day dresses or fantasy evening gowns.

It has been said that you are inspired by people such as Marie Antoinette and by eighteenth-century French art (France again). Can you tell me what it is about the two that has inspired you? In my opinion, literature, architecture, music, art and fashion peaked at the end of the eighteenth century. I love the beauty, the opulence, the frivolity and the warmth of that period in time.

What are you currently working on? I'm working on our latest collection as well as drawing for various private customers. We're also in the process of moving into our new offices … surprisingly, built in the eighteenth century. Also we are expanding the YDE brand internationally, which is very exciting.

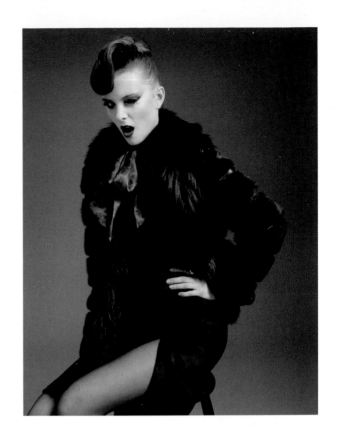

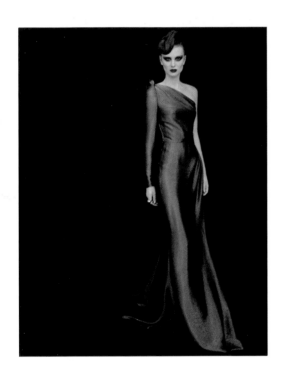

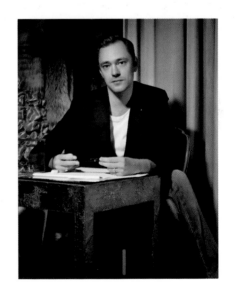

<u>Right:</u> Designer Ole Yde.

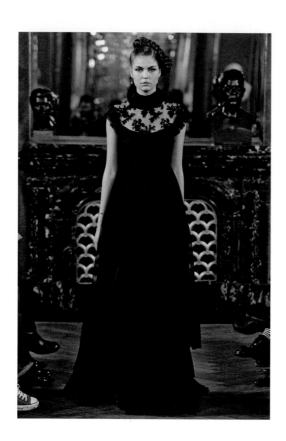

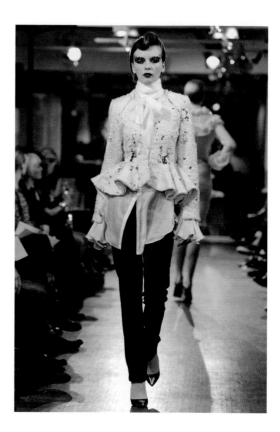

Opposite: Illustration by Ole Yde.

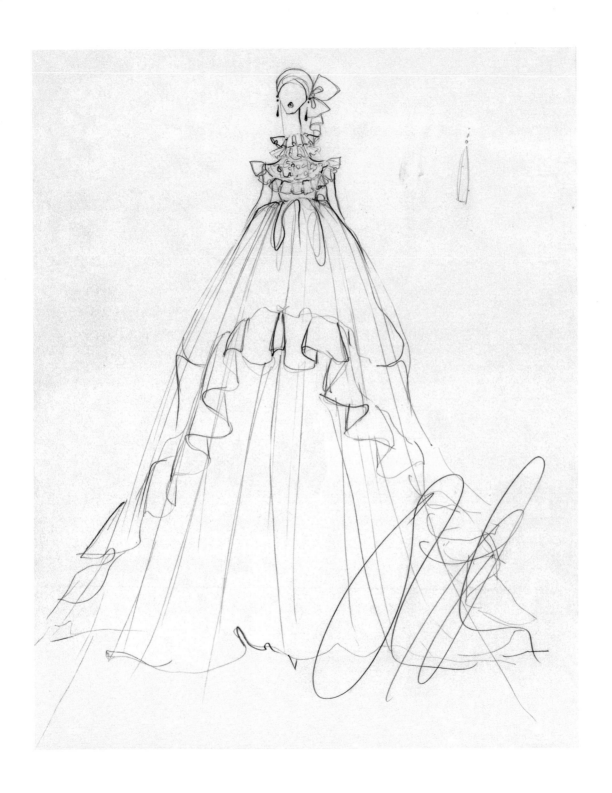

DIRECTORY

5PREVIEW
www.5preview.com

ACNE
www.acnestudios.com

ALTEWAI.SAOME
www.altewaisaome.com

ANN-SOFIE BACK
http://annsofieback.com

ANNE SOFIE MADSEN
www.annesofiemadsen.com

ASGER JUEL LARSEN
www.asgerjuellarsen.com

ASTRID ANDERSEN
www.astridandersen.com

BEATE GODAGER
www.beategodager.com

BRUUNS BAZAAR
www.bruunsbazaar.dk

BY MALENE BIRGER
www.bymalenebirger.com

CAMILLA STÆRK
www.staerk.com

CARIN WESTER
www.carinwester.com

COS
www.cosstores.com

DAY BIRGER ET MIKKELSEN
www.day.dk

DESIGNERS REMIX
www.designersremix.com

EYGLÓ
http://eyglocollection.com

V AVE SHOE REPAIR
www.vave-shoerepair.com

FILIPPA K
www.filippa-k.com

GAIA
http://gaiabrandt.com

HAANING & HTOON
www.haaningandhtoon.com

HEIKKI SALONEN
www.heikkisalonen.com

HENRIK VIBSKOV
www.henrikvibskov.com

HOPE
www.hope-sthlm.com

HOUSE OF DAGMAR
www.houseofdagmar.se

IDA SJÖSTEDT
www.idasjostedt.com

IVAN GRUNDAHL
www.ivangrundahl.dk

IVANA HELSINKI
www.ivanahelsinki.com

J.LINDEBERG
www.jlindeberg.com

JEAN PHILLIP
www.jeanphillip.dk

JOHANNA PIHL
www.johannapihl.com

KALDA
www.kalda.com

KRISTIAN AADNEVIK
www.kristianaadnevik.com

KRISTOFER KONGSHAUG
www.kristoferkongshaug.com

LIBERTINE-LIBERTINE
www.libertine-libertine.com

LOUISE SIGVARDT
www.louisesigvardt.dk

MARIA NORDSTRÖM
www.marianordstrom.com

MARIMEKKO
www.marimekko.fi

MINIMARKET
www.minimarket.se

MOONSPOON SALOON
www.moonspoonsaloon.tumblr.com

MUNDI
www.mundivondi.net

PETER JENSEN
www.peterjensen.co.uk

R/H
www.rh-the-label.com

RIIS
www.stineriis.com

RÜTZOU
www.rutzou.com

SAMUJI
www.samuji.com

SANDRA BACKLUND
www.sandrabacklund.com

SOULLAND
www.soulland.eu

SPON DIOGO
www.spondiogo.com

STINE GOYA
www.stinegoya.com

TIGER OF SWEDEN
www.tigerofsweden.com

VERONICA B. VALLENES
www.veronicabvallenes.com

VILSBØL DE ARCE
www.vilsboldearce.com

WEEKDAY
www.weekday.se

WHYRED
www.whyred.se

WOOD WOOD
www.woodwood.dk

YDE BY OLE YDE
www.yde-copenhagen.com

PICTURE CREDITS

p. 2 Photo by Sasha Maric.
p. 7 Photo by Nikolaj Møller.

5PREVIEW
p. 9 Photos of Linda Rodin by PAMU, Murray Hall and Paola Ambrosi; photo of Ragnar Persson courtesy 5PREVIEW studio.
p. 10 SS12 campaign (above left) by Fredrik Ottosson; catalogue (above right) shot by 2MANYPHOTOGRAPHERS; photos (below left and below right) by Natalia Aydin.
p. 11 Stills of Mieze Katz/MIA/Berlin from the video 'Fallschirm'; other photos courtesy 5PREVIEW studio.

ACNE
p. 13 Backstage photo by acnestudios.com.
p. 14 Photos by acnestudios.com.
p. 15 Photos by acnestudios.com.

ALTEWAI.SAOME
p. 16 Runway photo courtesy Mercedes Benz Fashion Week SS12; other photos courtesy Altewai Saome.
p. 17 Designer portrait by Karolina Krupa; other photos courtesy Altewai Saome.
p. 18 Campaign photos (above left and below right) by Alexander Dahl; lookbook photos (above right and below left) by Per Zennström.
p. 19 Campaign photo by Alexander Dahl.

ANN-SOFIE BACK
pp. 21–23 Photos by Dorothea Gundtoft.

ANNE SOFIE MADSEN
p. 25 Campaign photo by Hans Zeuthen.
p. 26 Lookbook and campaign photos by Hans Zeuthen; runway photos by Dorothea Gundtoft.
p. 28 Lookbook photos by Hans Zeuthen; illustration by Anne Sofie Madsen.
p. 29 Illustration by Anne Sofie Madsen.

ASGER JUEL LARSEN
p. 30 Campaign SS12 photo by Jens Stoltze; New York campaign photo (below left) by Andras Ridovics.
pp. 30–31 Campaign SS12 photo by Jens Stoltze.
p. 31 Runway photo by Simon Armstrong.
p. 32 Copenhagen campaign photo by Jens Stoltze; lookbook photo (above right) by Ellis Scott.
pp. 32–33 New York campaign photo by Andras Ridovics.
p. 33 Runway photo by Simon Armstrong.

ASTRID ANDERSEN
p. 35 Photo by Ellis Scott.
p. 36 Runway photo courtesy London Fashion Week.
p. 37 Photos by Dorothea Gundtoft.

BEATE GODAGER
pp. 39–41 Photos by Amanda Hestehave.

BRUNS BAZAAR
p. 42 Runway photo by Helle Moos; exterior photo by Dorte Krogh; campaign photo by Henrik Bülow.
p. 43 Designer portrait by Christian Friis; runway photo by Helle Moos; interior photo by Dorte Krogh.
p. 44 Lookbook photos by Andreas Larsson.

BY MALENE BIRGER
p. 47 Runway photo by Helle Moos.
p. 48 Photos by Thomas Nielsen.
p. 50 Campaign photo by Noam Griegst.
p. 51 Photos from Malene Birger book by Christian Burmeister; showroom photo by Dorothea Gundtoft; shop interior photo by Malene Birger In-House; runway photo by Helle Moos.

CAMILLA STÆRK
p. 53 Runway photo by Dan Lecca.
p. 54 Stills by Barnaby Roper.

CARIN WESTER
p. 56 Backstage photos by Sonny Vandevelde; lookbook photo (above right) by Fredrik Skogkvist; showroom photo (below left) by Dave Lau.
pp. 56–57 Black and white backstage photo by Lasse Bak Mejlvang; show image by Salvatore Scappini.
p. 57 Backstage photos by Sonny Vandevelde.
p. 59 Runway photos by Kristian Löveborg.

COS
p. 61 Campaign photo by Willy Vanderperre.
p. 62 Table setting photo courtesy of COS; campaign photos by Willy Vanderperre.
pp. 62–63 Photo courtesy of COS.
p. 63 Campaign photo (above left) by Willy Vanderperre; shop interior photos courtesy of COS; lookbook photo (below right) by Aitken Jolly.

DAY BIRGER ET MIKKELSEN
p. 64 Campaign photo by Frederik Jacobi; DAY Birger et Mikkelsen Home photo by Ditte Isager; runway photo courtesy DAY Birger et Mikkelsen
pp. 64–65 Campaign photo by Frederik Jacobi.
p. 65 Black and white campaign photo by Noam Griegst.
p. 66 Campaign photos by Noam Griegst; interior photos (below left and below right) by Ditte Isager.
p. 67 Campaign photo by Noam Griegst.

DESIGNERS REMIX
p. 69 Campaign photo by Jens Langkjær.
p. 70 Shop interior courtesy Designers Remix; campaign photos by Jens Langkjær; runway photo by Helle Moos.
pp. 70–71 Campaign photo by Jens Langkjær.
p. 71 Office interior courtesy Designers Remix; runway photo by Helle Moos.
pp. 72–73 Backstage photo by Katrine Rohrberg.

EYGLO
p. 75 Show image (above right) by www.lastnights-party.com; other photos courtesy EYGLO.
p. 76 Campaign photo by Arnold Björnsson.
p. 77 Lookbook photo (right) by Ester Ir; other photos courtesy EYGLO.

V AVE SHOE REPAIR
p. 79 Campaign photo by Nils Odier.
p. 80 Runway photo by Mattias Lindbäck; campaign photo by Nils Odier.
p. 81 Campaign photo by Nils Odier.

FILIPPA K
p. 83 Campaign photos by Alasdair McLellan; other photos courtesy Filippa K.
p. 84 Black and white photo by David Sims; other photos courtesy Filippa K.
p. 85 Campaign photo by Alasdair McLellan.

GAIA
p. 87 Collages by Gaia; campaign photo by Louise Damgaard.
p. 88 Runway photos by Brian Buchard; backstage photo by Louise Damgaard.
p. 89 Lookbook photo by Louise Damgaard.

HAANING & HTOON
p. 90 Campaign photo by Suzanne Emanuelsson; other photos by Min Htoon.
pp. 90–91 Photo by Min Htoon.
p. 91 Lookbook behind-the-scenes photo by Min Htoon.
p. 92 Showroom photo by Min Htoon; campaign photo by Suzanne Emanuelsson.
p. 93 Campaign photo by Tove Sivertsen.

HEIKKI SALONEN
p. 94 Runway photo by Chris Moore; campaign photo by Nicole Maria Winkler.
pp. 94–95 Campaign photo by Johanna Eliisa Laitanen.
p. 95 Campaign photo by Johanna Eliisa Laitanen.
p. 96 Campaign photos (left and above right) by Nicole Maria Winkler; campaign photo (below right) by Johanna Eliisa Laitanen.
p. 97 Campaign photo by Johanna Eliisa Laitanen.

HENRIK VIBSKOV
p. 98 Campaign photo by HV Studio; installation photo by Alastair Philip Wiper.
pp. 98–99 'The Shrink Wrap Spectacular' AW12 show image by Dorothea Gundtoft.
p. 99 Designer portrait by Dorothea Gundtoft; 'The Eat' AW11 show image by Alastair Philip Wiper.
pp. 100–101 'The Fantabulous Bicycle Music Factory' SS08 collection photos by Alastair Philip Wiper.
p. 102 Interior photos by Alastair Philip Wiper; runway photos by Dorothea Gundtoft.
p. 103 Runway photo courtesy Copenhagen Fashion Week.

PICTURE CREDITS

HOPE
p. 105 Photo courtesy Hope.
p. 106 Photos courtesy Hope.
p. 107 Runway and lookbook photos courtesy Hope.

HOUSE OF DAGMAR
p. 109 Backstage photo by Viktor Gårdsäter.
p. 110 Interior photo by Dagmar; lookbook photo and designer portrait by Pierre Björk.
p. 111 Runway photo (above left) by Dorothea Gundtoft; runway photo (above right) by Kristian Löveborg; photo (below right) by Viktor Gårdsäter; backstage photo of designer Giulia at work (bottom) by Sonny Photos.

IDA SJÖSTEDT
p. 113 Campaign photo by Ceen Wahren.
p. 114 Campaign photo by Ceen Wahren.
p. 115 Photos by Hedvig Jenning.

IVAN GRUNDAHL
p. 116 Campaign photo by Nicky de Silva; office interior photo by Ausa Thorvardarson; shop interior by Marc Kjelmann.
p. 117 Campaign photos by Nicky De Silva.

IVANA HELSINKI
p. 119 Runway photo by Filippo Fiore.
pp. 120–23 All photos courtesy Ivana Helsinki Studio.

J.LINDEBERG
p. 125 Campaign photo by Jörgen Ringstrand/model William Eustace, Success Models Paris.
p. 126 Runway photo (above left) by Kristian Löveborg; lookbook photo by Jörgen Ringstrand; bicycle photo by BikeID; runway photo (below right) by Kristian Löveborg/model Alexander Johansson, Elite Stockholm.
p. 127 Photo (above left) courtesy J.Lindeberg; product image (above right) by Jörgen Ringstrand; campaign photo (below left) by Andreas Sjödin/model Dorothea Barth Jörgensen, Elite Stockholm; photo (below right) courtesy J.Lindeberg.

JEAN PHILLIP
p. 129 Campaign photo by Hans Zeuthen.
p. 130 Backstage photos (below left and centre) by Dorothea Gundtoft; all other photos by Gert Foget Hansen.
p. 131 Backstage photo by Dorothea Gundtoft.

JOHANNA PIHL
pp. 132–35 Campaign photos by Patrick Lindblom.

KALDA
p. 137 Campaign photo by Silja Magg.
p. 138 Campaign photo (above left) by Silja Magg; interior photo (below) by Katrín Alda.
pp. 138–39 Photos by Katrín Alda.
p. 139 Lookbook photo by Silja Magg.

KRISTIAN AADNEVIK
p. 140 Sketch courtesy Kristian Aadnevik; backstage photo by Michelle Beatty; runway photo by Alex Barron-Hough.
pp. 140–41 Backstage photo by Michelle Beatty.
p. 141 Campaign photo by Chad Pickard & Paul McLean; runway photo by Alex Barron-Hough.
p. 142 Campaign photo by Chad Pickard & Paul McLean.
p. 143 Backstage photo by Michelle Beatty.

KRISTOFER KONGSHAUG
p. 145 Campaign photo by Timothy Elias Wright.
p. 146 Campaign photos (above and centre) by Hector Perez; photo (below) by Federico de Angelis.
p. 147 Campaign photo by Federico de Angelis.
pp. 148–49 Campaign photo by Hector Perez.

LIBERTINE-LIBERTINE
pp. 151–53 Photos by Sacha Maric.

LOUISE SIGVARDT
p. 155 Campaign photo by Sacha Maric.
p. 156 Campaign photos by Sacha Maric.
p. 157 Campaign photos by Sacha Maric; runway photos courtesy Copenhagen Fashion Week.
p. 158 Campaign photos by Sacha Maric.
p. 159 Campaign photo by Sacha Maric.

MARIA NORDSTRÖM
p. 161 Backstage photo by Frida Marklund.
p. 162 Backstage photo by Frida Marklund.
p. 163 Runway photo by Kristian Löveborg; other photos courtesy Maria Nordström.
p. 164 Campaign photo by Axel Lindahl.
p. 165 Campaign photos by Axel Lindahl; show image (above centre) by Dorothea Gundtoft; backstage photo (above right) by Frida Marklund; show image (below centre) by Mikael Olsson; sketch courtesy Maria Nordström.

MARIMEKKO
pp. 167–69 All photos courtesy Marimekko.

MINIMARKET
p. 171 Campaign photo by Peter Gehrke/Adamsky.
p. 172 Runway photo by Kristian Löveborg; other photos courtesy Minimarket.
p. 173 Lookbook photo by Peter Gehrke/Adamsky; other photos courtesy Minimarket.
p. 174 Runway photo by Kristian Löveborg.
p. 175 Runway photos by Kristian Löveborg; lookbook photos by Peter Gehrke/Adamsky.

MOONSPOON SALOON
p. 176 Lookbook (left) by Eliot Lee Hazel; campaign photo (below right) by Frederik Jacobi; ? drawing courtesy Tal R.
pp. 176–77 Lookbook behind-the-scenes photo by Sara Sachs.
p. 177 Campaign photo by Noam Griegst.

p. 178 Drawing courtesy Tal R.
p. 179 Show photos by Dorothea Gundtoft; designer portrait by Melanie Buchhave; product image by Sara Sachs.

MUNDI
p. 180 Campaign photo by Hürdur Sveinsson.
pp. 180–81 Photo by Thibault Pradet.
p. 181 Artwork courtesy Mundi; campaign photo by Fridrik Örn.
p. 182 Artwork courtesy 'Moms'; runway photos by Fridrik Örn.

PETER JENSEN
p. 185 Photo of Karen Elson and Peter Jensen by Tim Walker.
p. 186 Photos by Alexander Wilson.
p. 187 Photo (above) by Alexander Wilson; designer portrait (below) courtesy Peter Jensen.
p. 188 Photo (above left) courtesy Peter Jensen; backstage photo (above right) by Paul Bliss; campaign photo (below left) by Tina Barney; campaign photo with logo (below right) by Max Farago.
p. 189 Campaign photo by Jane Mcleish-Kelsey.

R/H
p. 191 Image (above left) courtesy R/H; lookbook photo (above right) by Karoliina Bärlund; photo (below) by Juuso Westerlund.
p. 193 Photo (above left) courtesy R/H; designer portrait (above right) by Rami Lappalainen; campaign photo (centre right) by Karoliina Bärlund; sketch (below left) courtesy R/H; shop interior (below right) courtesy R/H.

RIIS
p. 195 Campaign photo by Hill & Aubrey.
p. 196 Lookbook photo by Stine Riis and Avon Bashida; runway photo courtesy H&M Design Awards; designer portrait by Sara Galbiati.
p. 197 Notebooks courtesy Stine Riis; runway photo courtesy H&M Design Awards.

RÜTZOU
p. 199 Campaign photo by Henrik Bülow.
p. 201 Designer portrait by Sascha Oda; lookbook photo by Sascha Oda; runway photo by Sacha Maric; campaign photo by Henrik Bülow.

SAMUJI
pp. 202–205 Campaign photo by Juliana Harkki; all other photos by Ville Varumo.

SANDRA BACKLUND
p. 207 Campaign photo by Peter Gehrke.
p. 208 Campaign photos by Thomas Klementsson; product image (above right) by Kristian Löveborg; photo (below left) by Kristian Bengtsson.
p. 209 Campaign photo by Thomas Klementsson.

PICTURE CREDITS

SOULLAND

p. 211 Lookbook photo by Nikolaj Møller.

p. 212 Backstage photo (above left) by Sascha Oda; photo (above right) courtesy Soulland; photo of hatmaker's workshop (below) by Nikolaj Møller.

pp. 212–13 Backstage photo by Sascha Oda.

p. 213 Campaign photo by Nikolaj Møller; backstage photo by Sascha Oda.

p. 214 Lookbook photos by Nikolaj Møller; campaign photos by Nikolaj Møller.

SPON DIOGO

p. 217 Lookbook photo by Alfredo Salazar.

p. 218 Runway photo by Michael Hermansen; campaign photo by Isa Jacob.

p. 219 Backstage photo by Dorothea Gundtoft; campaign photo by Nikolaj Møller; designer portrait by Michael Hermansen.

STINE GOYA

p. 221 Campaign photo by Casper Sejersen.

p. 222 Campaign photo by Casper Sejersen; runway photo courtesy Copenhagen Fashion Week; other photos courtesy Stine Goya.

p. 223 Runway photo (above left) by Sacha Maric; backstage photo (above right) by Jonas Hoejgaard; backstage photo (below left) by Dorothea Gundtoft; designer portrait by Rasmus B. Lind.

TIGER OF SWEDEN

p. 225 Campaign photos by Hans Nielsen; portrait by David.

p. 226 Campaign photos by Hans Nielsen; photo (below left) by Joel Rodin.

p. 227 Interior photo courtesy Tiger of Sweden.

VERONICA B. VALLENES

p. 228 Runway photo courtesy Copenhagen Fashion Week; studio photo courtesy Veronica B. Vallenes.

pp. 228–29 Studio photo courtesy Veronica B. Vallenes.

p. 229 Runway photo courtesy Copenhagen Fashion Week.

p. 231 Campaign photos by Hans Zeuthen; runway photos courtesy Copenhagen Fashion Week.

VILSBØL DE ARCE

p. 232 Black and white photo (left) by Oliver Stalmans; campaign photo (above) by Nikolaj Møller.

pp. 232–33 Campaign photo by Nikolaj Møller.

p. 233 Runway photo by Anders Hviid; campaign photo (below) by Nikolaj Møller.

p. 234 Campaign photo (left) by Oliver Stalmans; campaign photo (right) by Nikolaj Holm Møller.

p. 235 Campaign photo by Nikolaj Holm Møller.

WEEKDAY

pp. 237–39 Photos courtesy Weekday.

WHYRED

pp. 241 Lookbook photo by Hannes Söderlund.

p. 242 Runway photos by Kristian Löveborg; shop exterior courtesy Whyred.

p. 243 Runway photos by Kristian Löveborg; product image courtesy Whyred.

WOOD WOOD

p. 245 Campaign photo (above) by Sacha Maric; photo (below left) courtesy Wood Wood; show image (below right) by Dorothea Gundtoft.

p. 246 Photo by Henrik Bülow.

pp. 246–47 Shop interior by Stamers Kontor.

p. 247 Product image courtesy Wood Wood; runway photo by Dorothea Gundtoft; shop interior by Stamers Kontor.

YDE BY OLE YDE

p. 249 Campaign photos and designer portrait by Asger Mortensen.

p. 250 Runway photos courtesy Copenhagen Fashion Week.

p. 251 Sketch courtesy Ole Yde.

ACKNOWLEDGMENTS

I would very much like to thank everyone who has
helped me through this project, from designers to editors
and the great team at Thames & Hudson – especially Jamie
Camplin for believing in me and this book. Lastly, I could not
have got through this without the neverending support of my
mother, the tough but honest advice of my father and
the kind hospitality of my grandmother.

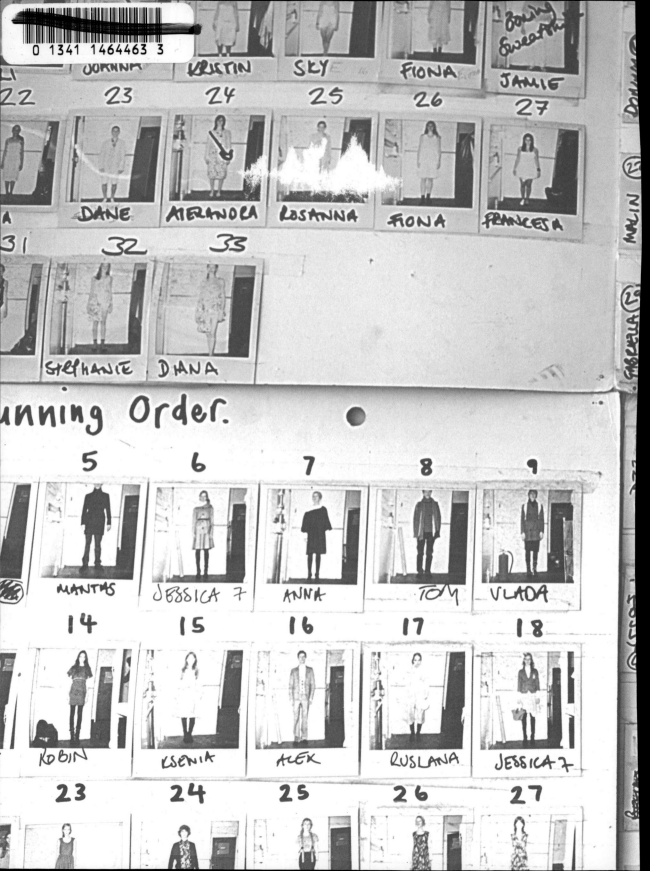

JORNNA 23   KRISTIN 24   SKY 25   FIONA 26   JAMIE 27

22

DANE   ALEXANDRA   ROSANNA   FIONA   FRANCESCA

31   32   33

STEPHANIE   DIANA

unning Order.

5   6   7   8   9

MANTAS   JESSICA 7   ANNA   TOM   VLADA

14   15   16   17   18

ROBIN   KSENIA   ALEK   RUSLANA   JESSICA 7

23   24   25   26   27